Disclaimer

Ketogenic Diet

Quick and Easy Cookbook Recipes and Meal Plans for Boosting Your Metabolism, Increasing Energy Levels, and Losing Weight

By Susan Hollister

Table of Contents

INTRODUCTION..8

WHERE IT STARTED 8
WHAT IS KETOSIS? 8
HOW THE DIET WORKS............................ 9
BENEFITS BEYOND WEIGHT LOSS 9
SETTING UP YOUR DIET PLAN OF SUCCESS 11
WHAT ARE MACROS?............................. 13
NET CARBOHYDRATES 13
PROTEIN AND FAT................................ 14
WHAT TO EXPECT IN KETOSIS 15
GEARING UP 16
MEDICAL OVERSIGHT MAY BE NEEDED 17
YOUR VERY OWN MACROS 17
LET YOUR BODY ADJUST........................ 17
YOUR CULINARY ADVENTURE 18

CHAPTER 1: KETO-FRIENDLY INGREDIENTS.............. 20

LOW-CARB THICKENING AGENTS 20
SEEDS 21
FLOUR-LIKE SUBSTANCES....................... 21
SWEETNESS WITHOUT THE SUGAR 25
SOURCES OF FIBER............................... 27
THE SCOOP ON POOP 27
SOURCES OF SOLUBLE FIBER (TO TREAT DIARRHEA): 28
SOURCES OF INSOLUBLE FIBER (TO TREAT CONSTIPATION): 28
OILS AND OTHER FATS.......................... 28
OTHER ATYPICAL INGREDIENTS 31

CHAPTER 2: DELICIOUS APPETIZERS 33

APPLE AND HAM FLATBREAD 33
BABA GANOUSH (EGGPLANT DIP) 35
BUFFALO CHICKEN STRIPS...................... 38
CHEESY SPINACH PUFFS 40
CHEESEBURGER MUFFINS 42
CHEESY SPINACH ROLLS WITH APPLE-SLAW TOPPING 45

GROUND CHICKEN MEATBALLS WITH KICK 48

LOW-CARB SESAME CRACKERS 50

SCOTCH EGGS.. 52

SPICY SMOKY HOT CRAB DIP 55

CHAPTER 3: SCRUMPTIOUS SALADS AND DRESSINGS. 58

CAULIFLOWER "POTATO" SALAD 58

FRESH CHICKEN SALAD 60

GREEK LEMON DRESSING... 63

LEMON-AVOCADO TUNA SALAD 64

LOW-CARB CREAMY RANCH DRESSING 65

STRAWBERRY VINAIGRETTE DRESSING 67

TAMARI STEAK SALAD 68

TURKEY ARUGULA SALAD.. 71

ZESTY LOW-CARB ITALIAN DRESSING 72

ZESTY TACO SALAD 74

CHAPTER 4: TASTY SOUPS AND STEWS...................... 76

BRAZILIAN SPICY FISH STEW (MOQUECA) 76

CHICKEN ZUCCHINI-NOODLE SOUP 78

COMFORTING CHICKEN CROCK-POT STEW 79

ECONOMICAL HAMBURGER VEGGIE SOUP....................................... 82

GOOD-FOR-YOU CREAM OF BROCCOLI SOUP.................................. 85

HEARTY BEEF STEW 87

NOODLE-LESS CHICKEN SOUP 90

PORK CHILI VERDI (GREEN CHILI PORK STEW) 92

PUMPKIN-PORK STEW À LA CROCK-POT 94

RICH, HEART-WARMING TOMATO SOUP 96

CHAPTER 5: BEEF RECIPES THAT WILL MAKE YOUR MOUTH WATER 100

BEEF STROGANOFF WITH ZUCCHINI NOODLES 100

CHEESE-STUFFED BACON BURGERS 102

CROCK-POT BEEF POT ROAST.. 105

GREEK-INSPIRED BEEF ZUCCHINI BURGERS................................... 108

GREEN BEAN AND HAMBURGER SKILLET.. 109

KETO ROASTED BRISKET 111

KETOGENIC STEAK 113

SESAME BEEF AND DAIKON STIR FRY 116

SLOW-COOKED BEEF AND BROCCOLI STIR FRY................................. 119

STEAK PINWHEELS.. 121

CHAPTER 6: WORLD CLASS POULTRY RECIPES 125

BREADED PARMESAN BACON CHICKEN.. 125

CHICKEN PARMESAN CASSEROLE 128

JUICY LEMON PEPPER CHICKEN 131

KETOGENIC CHICKEN ALFREDO CASSEROLE................................... 133

LOW-CARB TURKEY TETRAZZINI 135

NOT-SO-OLD-FASHIONED TURKEY POT PIE..................................... 138

PAN-SEARED DUCK À L'ORANGE OVER WILTED SPINACH................... 141

SIMPLY SMASHING STUFFED CHICKEN ROLLS 143

SLOW-COOKED CHICKEN COCONUT CURRY 146

CHAPTER 7: PORK RECIPES FIT FOR ROYALTY 148

ANYTIME CRANBERRY-APRICOT-GLAZED BAKED HAM........................ 148

ASIAN PORK CHOPS 150

BACON-WRAPPED PORK ROAST.. 153

BALSAMIC ROAST TENDERLOIN A LA CROCK-POT 157

BOURBON-GLAZED HAM 158

HOLIDAY-WORTHY CRISPY ROAST PORK LEG 160

PARMESAN PORK CHOPS 163

PORK AND VEGGIE STIR FRY.. 165

PORK CHOPS WITH VELVETY GRAVY 167

PULLED PORK 170

CHAPTER 8: TENDER AND TASTY LOW-CARB LAMB.. 173

CROCK-POT LAMB ROAST 173

EXOTIC LAMB CURRY WITH SPINACH (SAAG GOSHT) 175

GREEK LAMB BURGERS WITH MINT 177

ITALIAN LAMB CHOPS WITH FRESH PESTO 179

MOROCCAN LAMB CHOPS 182

NOT-SO-IRISH LAMB STEW.. 184

PAN-SEARED LAMB CHOPS IN MUSTARD SAUCE 186

ROAST LEG OF LAMB 189

TENDER LAMB SHANKS À LA CROCK POT 191

TURKISH LAMB WITH LOW-CARB PITA... 193

CHAPTER 9: MELT IN YOUR MOUTH SEAFOOD DISHES

.... **198**

BACON AND SHRIMP 198

CAULIFLOWER FISH CAKES WITH AIOLI.............................. 199

CHEESY BAKED SEA SCALLOPS... 202

CLAM CHOWDER À LA CROCK-POT 205

FUSS-FREE FOIL-BAKED HALIBUT 208

KETO FISH NUGGETS.. 209

KETO SHRIMP SCAMPI.. 212

LOW-CARB – YES, IT IS POSSIBLE – LOBSTER ROLL 214

PAN-SEARED BUTTER SALMON 215

SUPER SIMPLE CRAB VEGETABLE OMELET CASSEROLE 218

CHAPTER 10: SIDES AND SAUCES............................ **220**

AIOLI 220

FAUX MACARONI AND CHEESE 221

FAUX MASHED POTATOES 223

FAUX RICE, A.K.A., RICED CAULIFLOWER............................ 225

FAUX TATER TOTS 228

FRIED GREEN BEANS.. 229

HOT ASIAN BROCCOLI SALAD 232

HOW TO COOK SPAGHETTI SQUASH 234

KETO BUNS.. 235

KETO GRAVY 237

KETO-APPROVED KETCHUP 238

KETO-APPROVED SAUSAGE GRAVY (COUNTRY GRAVY)....... 240

KETOGENIC BREAD 242

KETOGENIC MAYONNAISE 243

LOW-CARB TORTILLAS... 245

NUTTY ROASTED GREEN BEANS 247

PESTO... 249

PSEUDO WILD RICE MUSHROOM PILAF............................. 250

TWICE-BAKED ZUCCHINI 252

ZOODLES – THE VERSATILE ZUCCHINI NOODLE................ 254

ZUCCHINI PARMESAN FRIES... 259

CHAPTER 11: EASY MEAL PLANS............................ **261**

WHERE TO START 261
WATCH YOUR INGREDIENTS 262
BEEF-LOVER'S MEAL #1 263
BEEF-LOVER'S MEAL #2 263
BEEF-LOVER'S MEAL #3 264
POULTRY-LOVER'S MEAL #1 264
POULTRY-LOVER'S MEAL #2 264
PORK-LOVER'S MEAL #1 265
PORK-LOVER'S MEAL #2 265
LAMB-LOVER'S MEAL #1 265
LAMB-LOVER'S MEAL #2 265
FISH WITH ASPARAGUS 266
SHRIMP-LOVER'S MEAL 266
FISH-LOVER'S MEAL 266

CONCLUSION 268
MY OTHER BOOKS... 270

Introduction

Congratulations on purchasing this book. You have made a wise decision. In these pages are a large variety of delicious recipes that you can use to become a healthy fat burning machine.

The ketogenic diet is a low-carb, high-protein diet that can generate great changes in how your body acquires energy and burns fat. This diet is well-known for promoting weight loss, lowering cholesterol and reducing blood pressure. It has also been found to enhance memory, improve acne and help stabilize blood sugar levels along with a variety of other benefits.

Where It Started

The ketogenic diet developed because the son of a Hollywood producer was stricken with epilepsy. The seizures were frequent and violent, prompting Jim Abrahams – the desperate father – to embark on a search for any effective treatment. When nothing they tried had any noticeable effect, Mr. Abrahams delved into existing research, hoping to find something that would help his son.

He eventually came across a book on epilepsy, written by Dr. John Freeman, who proposed specific dietary restrictions as a treatment. The proposed diet was low in carbohydrates and high in protein. It was based on a 1920s diet that involved fasting. When a person fasts, the body produces a substance known as ketones, which help to minimize seizures. The Freeman diet apparently fools the body into thinking it is fasting, which triggers the production of ketones.

What Is Ketosis?

Ketosis is a physical state in which the body relies on ketones for energy. These ketones are produced by the liver, as it breaks down fats. Normally, our energy is derived from blood sugar. Carbohydrates are converted to sugar. Insulin then kicks in to process the sugar that is circulating in our bloodstream. However, when carbohydrates are removed from the diet, their absence encourages the body to turn to the fat in your food and the fat stored in your body to produce ketones. These ketones are then "burned" to produce the energy you need to keep your body going. Once your body is relying on ketones for energy production you are said to be in ketosis.

How The Diet Works

The objective of the ketogenic diet is to trigger ketosis and keep your body functioning in this state. This is accomplished by limiting the intake of carbohydrates while increasing protein and fat consumption. This keeps blood glucose at healthy levels. Instead of producing insulin to deal with all the glucose, the body switches over, allowing the liver to break down fats and create ketones. In the process, your body starts to burn its existing fat stores.

Benefits Beyond Weight Loss

- **Lower Blood Sugar** - The type of foods in the ketogenic diet tend to keep blood sugar levels lower and more stable. The diet works well for many Type II diabetics. If you have diabetes, this diet should be implemented under close medical supervision.

- **Mental Performance** – Many people report increased mental alertness on this diet. There is evidence to suggest that a ketogenic diet may boost memory skills, creativity, reasoning, and thought clarity. Because it stabilizes the blood sugar – preventing the wild swings between high and low – it makes sense that your focus and concentration would improve.

- **More Energy** – Ketones are the most effective source of energy; consequently, most people feel invigorated while on this diet. Evidence strongly indicates that fat burning is the most efficient form of energy production in the body; the ketogenic diet capitalizes on this truth.

- **Fewer Hunger Pangs** – A high-fat, high-protein diet satisfies hunger pangs more effectively than carbs and sugars. It is quite normal to go through a day without feeling hungry while on this diet.

- **Blood Pressure and Cholesterol** – in many people, blood pressure and cholesterol levels drop, often quite dramatically. In some studies, the ketogenic diet was reported to drastically increase HDL and decrease LDL cholesterol levels. Common wisdom says that eating fat is bad for you, but that's not true when your body is burning it for energy.

- **Insulin Resistance** – This is often the precursor to full-blown diabetes. Because sugar levels are stabilized by this diet, insulin resistance is often reduced and diabetes can be averted.

- **Acne** – All sorts of inflammations are reduced by the ketogenic diet. Carbohydrates can exacerbate inflammation throughout the body, so it stands to reason that if you eat fewer carbohydrates, all sorts of inflammation would be reduced. Since acne is a form of inflammation, you can expect to see less of it over the course of this diet.

- **Epilepsy** – I am *not* touting the ketogenic diet as a cure, but it came into existence because it was found effective at reducing seizures. If you are living with epilepsy, I suggest that you explore the possibility of using this diet, under the direct supervision of a physician, of course.

Setting Up Your Diet Plan of Success

The Ketogenic diet takes a little bit of preparation to get started on it properly, but this small amount of time and effort will be well spent when you start seeing the incredible results this diet can offer. Ideally you want to know specifically how much of the essential nutrients you need. You'll be tracking the amount of fat, protein, and carbohydrates you take in with each meal. This diet is quite restrictive, limiting you to as few as 15 grams of carbohydrate per day. That's not very much. We're talking a single slice of bread, a tablespoon of sugar, a small apple, or a cup of milk. But the increase to your overall health and wellbeing is so worth it when you do things correctly.

The ketogenic diet uses vegetables, nuts, and dairy as carbohydrate sources and avoids *all* processed carbohydrates, including bread, pasta, cereal, potatoes, beans, and most fruit. Grains and sugar are things you definitely want to avoid if you truly want to get the best benefits of this diet.

Meats of all varieties are encouraged. Any vegetable grown above ground is good, as are nuts and seeds. Cheeses make up a hefty part of the diet and fats like coconut oil, high-fat salad dressings, and saturated fats are considered okay. The only fruits suggested are berries, because they are low-glycemic.

Drinks can be an issue, but water, coffee, and tea are quite acceptable with this diet, as long as they aren't sugared.

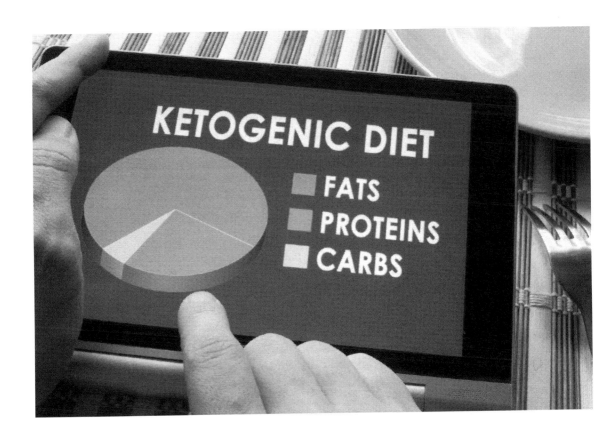

This diet does not count calories; instead it counts grams related to three key nutritional categories. In most cases, your nutrient consumption should be broken down into about 70% fats, 25% protein, and 5% carbohydrates. This is not always easy to balance. The fewer carbohydrates you take in, the more weight you will lose, but do not get carried away and cut them out entirely; your body actually needs the nutrients available in carbohydrates – just not as much of them as you're currently getting.

It's to start the diet all at one time without easing into it. At the same time, you can start at a basic level and give your body time to adjust to the new diet. Once your body has shifted into the state of ketosis and is stable there, then you will be able to tweak your diet to help you maintain good energy levels while losing or maintaining weight.

The recipes in this book will give you a convenient table so you can easily see what you can eat and how much. The nutritional information is very easy to understand and use so so you can easily calculate what foods and recipes to eat for the day.

What Are Macros?

The term "macros" is short for "macronutrients" and will be the primary form of measurement you will use to develop meal plans and draw up menus. Specifically, the term refers to the amount of fat, carbohydrates, and protein your body requires to function optimally when in ketosis. You'll use these numbers to balance your nutritional needs throughout the day.

Each of the recipes in this book is introduced with a table that provides everything you need to know about its nutritional content. For example, here is the nutritional table for broccoli, a common ingredient in ketogenic meals:

Nutritional Information Per Serving			
Yield:	1 serving	Serving Size:	1 cup
Calories:	31	Fat:	0.3 grams
Carbohydrates:	6 grams	Protein:	2.6 grams
Fiber:	2.4 grams		

The nutritional information for raw broccoli

Net Carbohydrates

Carbohydrates will make up less than 5% of your total calories. In the nutritional tables provided in this book, the carbohydrates listed in the nutritional tables are the *total carbohydrates*. However, for this diet, you'll be tracking *net carbohydrates*. To calculate the net carbs in any of these recipes, you will subtract the amount of fiber from the provided total carbohydrates.

For example, one cup of broccoli (see the nutritional table, above) contains six grams of total carbohydrates. About 2.4 grams of that amount comes in the form of fiber, which is essential to proper digestion and shouldn't be counted as part of your daily carbohydrate intake. **To calculate the net carbohydrates**, you'll subtract the fiber (2.4 grams) from the total carbohydrates (6 grams) to get your net carbohydrate count of 3.6 grams in a cup of raw broccoli.

If you're used to counting calories, I have a little trick that may be of help. When it comes to calculating net carbohydrate intake, on average, there are 1.5 grams of net carbohydrates for every 100 calories. Of course, this is a very rough estimate, but it will help you get a general feel for this diet.

Protein And Fat

Protein and fat levels need to be measured and balanced, as well. Too much protein will prevent your body from shifting into ketosis, so your body can draw its energy from fat. Too little protein and your body won't have the energy it needs to function at its best. Your optimal protein intake for a day is 20% of your total diet. You can be a bit flexible between protein and fat amounts, but don't ever swap protein out for carbohydrates.

Your optimal level of protein consumption is dictated by your lean body mass. To calculate lean body mass, subtract your body fat percentage from your current weight. For most people, a moderate protein consumption level is between 0.06 grams and 1.2 grams per pound of lean body mass.

The key to balancing these components of your diet is to focus on getting enough fat each day. This is the most challenging part of this diet. After that, the other parts will fall into place.

A high fat level is desired, allowing you to produce energy when in ketosis. It causes you to feel full. This diet works best when you eat about 70% of your calories in higher fat meats like chicken thighs or legs. This means you can enjoy butter, sour cream, or cheese on your vegetables and you'll find all sorts of ingenious ways to introduce various oils into your dishes. Yes, go ahead, enjoy your bacon!

The recipes in this book are designed specifically to help you discover new sources for those all-important macronutrients and help you to adjust your lifestyle to support ketosis. As with anything new, it will require some conscious attention on your part in the beginning, but as you become accustomed to this new way of living your skills and proficiency will become second-nature and you will be amazed at how the fat comes off, your energy levels rise and the lack of hunger while on this diet.

What To Expect in Ketosis

You know when your body has attained ketosis when:

- You urinate more frequently.

- You have a dry mouth. Drink more water when this happens.

- You have bad breath. Ketones produce acetone, which smells like ripe fruit or nail polish remover. Eventually, this will go away. In the meanwhile, you can minimize the odor by brushing your teeth often, using mouthwash or by chewing sugar-free gum.

- You will be less hungry and more energized – at first you might not feel very good. While your body is adjusting to the change in diet you may actually feel ill and in a mental fog. This is a state that has been dubbed the "keto flu." Fortunately, this won't last long. Once you get beyond this point, your energy should pick up again and your thoughts should clear.

- Your mind is clear and focused. Once your body is in ketosis, your brain is burning ketones for energy, a much more efficient source than sugar. It leaves your mind free to think clearly.

- Insomnia is also a potential side effect, but it is temporary and serves as a sign that your body is adjusting to the new diet.

Alright, if you *really* want to know if your body is functioning ketogenically, there's a urine test you can run that will give you a general idea. You can purchase ketone test strips in many drug stores that will tell you how many ketones your body is producing. The strips are inexpensive and give you a general idea of how your body is doing. Over time, you should be able to use changes in ketone levels to adjust your diet. Blood tests are also available, but the urine test is simplest for the average person to use.

Gearing Up

Unless you've tried the Atkins diet, a form of ketogenic diet, you'll find this is nothing like other forms of dieting. It takes some planning to start off and you don't want to go gradually in either. If you are not serious about this diet, it will not give you the desired benefits and it can do damage to your body if you don't pay attention to what you are doing.

I have a friend who landed in the hospital on life support, because the diet was just too much for her to manage. She had ended up eating almost nothing, mostly because she didn't carve out time from her extremely busy schedule to plan meals that allowed her to take the proper foods to work with her.

This is not to scare you away from the diet; I just want to underscore that this is a very powerful process and as such can wreak some major havoc on your body if not properly administered and managed with care. By its very nature, the ketogenic diet is a long-term venture. It takes time to attain the state of ketosis and must be sustained for a long time to experience the health benefits you are looking for.

Medical Oversight May Be Needed

You are changing not only the way you eat, but the way your body processes energy; so if you have any doubts or health concerns, be sure to consult your doctor first about this diet. It is always nice to you have your doctor fully informed so they know how to identify potential danger signs, test for them, and treat them.

Your Very Own Macros

The next step in your preparation is to calculate your macronutrient levels. Each person's macros are different. You can't just make up any old plan randomly; you must calculate your macro values before you can effectively design any part of this diet.

The process of determining your macronutrient levels is fairly straightforward, but it involves several calculations. Before you get started, you need to know a couple key numbers. You need to know your weight; that should be simple enough to determine. Almost as easy, you need a rough estimate of your body fat percentage. If you don't know it already, you can search online for "body fat percentage pictures" and choose the percentage that looks most like the shape of your body. Your numbers will be good enough if your body fat percentage is within 30 percent accuracy.

Armed with these two numbers, search online for a macronutrient calculator and follow the instructions. For example, www.ketoconnect.net/calculator/ will walk you, step-by-step, through the process. You'll plug in the numbers and the calculator will provide the precise amount of each key nutrient necessary to maintain your current weight or drop pounds.

Let Your Body Adjust

Don't overdo things. Start by giving yourself 20 grams of daily carbohydrates for the first month, just until you get used to the diet. As your body becomes adjusted, you can gradually reduce the carbohydrate levels until you're maintaining your weight. Then, if you want to lose weight, you can further lower your carbohydrate intake a little more.

The keto flu can hit anytime during the first five to seven days. It is so-named because your body can feel like it's fighting a flu bug; you can feel tired, groggy, nauseous, and just generally under the weather. This isn't a genuine flu; it's just a sign your body is getting rid of excess sugar and other toxins. Your digestive system is also adjusting to processing different levels of fat than before, so you can expect diarrhea or constipation...or both, to appear as your body gets used to the new foods. Most of these symptoms, however, will diminish throughout the first month on the diet.

Avoid a strict reduction of calories for the first few weeks. Your body will have enough to handle while adjusting to the reduction in carbohydrates. Calorie reduction can wait until you're a month into the plan.

My best suggestion is to figure out what percentage of fats, carbs, and proteins are best for you through trial and error. A food journal is great for this. These recipes indicate the nutritional load per serving, so take advantage of them when making up your meal plans. Most importantly, once you've come up with a plan, stick to it.

Your Culinary Adventure

Because I'm taking away your bread and pasta and adding protein and fat to your diet, the least I could do is help you find reasonable substitutes for them. This process involves expanding your list of common ingredients to include items you may have never heard of before. You'll also discover ways to use well-known ingredients that you may not have imagined yet.

Also included in this book is advice on food substitutions, showing alternatives for other popular foods. This will equip you for using your own favorite recipes that may otherwise have too many carbohydrates, allowing you to substitute keto-friendly alternatives.

Before we delve into the recipes themselves, let's take a look at some of the exotic and healthy ingredients that you can add to your recipes.

Chapter 1: Keto-Friendly Ingredients

Here's a run-down of some of the more unusual ingredients you will encounter in ketogenic recipes, along with the part they play in promoting ketosis.

Low-Carb Thickening Agents

- Guar gum – can be used as a thickener in place of cornstarch. It also works well in conjunction with gluten-free flours in baking, helping to add some bounce and crispness to muffins, breads, and other baked goods. It can be added to liquids to help them mix more smoothly with other substances and can prevent oils from separating out. Use in moderation, as massive doses can swell up to block the intestines or the esophagus and have been reported to contribute to heart problems.

- Xanthum Gum – An excellent thickening agent. Many people use a 50-50 mix of guar and xanthum gums and report results that this combination is more effective than using either one by itself.

- Cream – Whipped and folded into soups, sauces, and puddings, this can thicken while adding that richness only cream can provide.

- Sour cream – I first learned to love sour cream, dollopped atop Ukrainian borscht. Now I use it on or in soups and as a thickener for gravies and savory sauces.

- Coconut flour – Mix one part coconut flour with one part water, then whisk into any hot liquid and stir until thickened to your liking.

- Ground chia seeds – Chia seeds are a wonderful low-carbohydrate substance with some pretty amazing properties. They absorb something like 11 times their weight in liquid, so you'll want to drink plenty of water if you eat them dry or toasted. In fact, the whole seeds are usually soaked in water for at least 5 minutes before using in recipes; otherwise they can swell inside you, dehydrating your body, and creating some uncomfortable sensations while they are being digested.

As a thickener for sauces, soups, or gravy, gradually stir in either the whole seeds or the ground powder, a little at a time, until you've reached the desired consistency.

Seeds

- Flax seeds – You can sprinkle the whole seeds on top of baked goods, in yogurt, or salads to add nutty crunch. The ground meal allows your body to absorb even more of the seed's nutrients. Use the meal in baked goods; it works well in muffins, as an extender for meatloaf. Note: if you're on a blood-thinner, you should avoid flax, as it can thin your blood even more.

  Flax meal can serve as an egg substitute in pancakes and cookies. In place of one egg, add one tablespoon of ground flax to three tablespoons of water and let it set for a couple of minutes before mixing it into your batter.

- Chia seeds – Used whole, these can be sprinkled atop salads and casseroles for a colorful, crunchy pop to your recipes. In baking, follow the instructions for using ground chia seeds, above

Flour-Like Substances

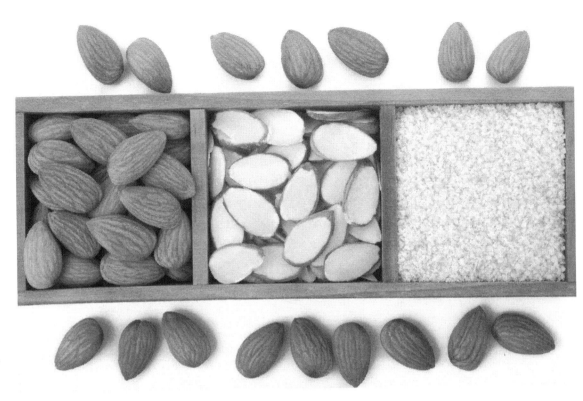

Almonds, left: whole, center: sliced, right: almond flour

- Almond flour – My favorite flour substitute. I mix it with almond meal, a more coarsely ground substance, for a nutty crunch in pie crust. In baking, you'll want to use it for no more than one fourth of the total flour content; any more, and your dough will crumble. In addition, you can offset the tendency to crumbliness by adding an extra egg to your mixture.

- Coconut flour – This is a close second to almond flour; besides, I like the flavor of coconut. To use in recipes, you'll want to add extra eggs and use less of it than regular flour. This flour absorbs more liquid than most of the flours you'll be using on this diet, but otherwise it will work well with your recipes.

- Egg white protein powder – Most of the time you'll be using the whole egg, since the yolk is full of the fat you're always looking to get in your diet. Egg whites, however, can stand in for the gluten you've removed when you nixed the carbs in wheat flour. Egg white powder can add some of the elasticity of gluten when you're making keto bread. Just keep in mind that the concentrated powder will add some protein to your diet.

- Sesame flour – Finely ground sesame seeds make a flour that is very close to wheat flour in texture and function. You'll want to mix sesame flour with psyllium flour in your baking if you want to rival the light texture of high-carb

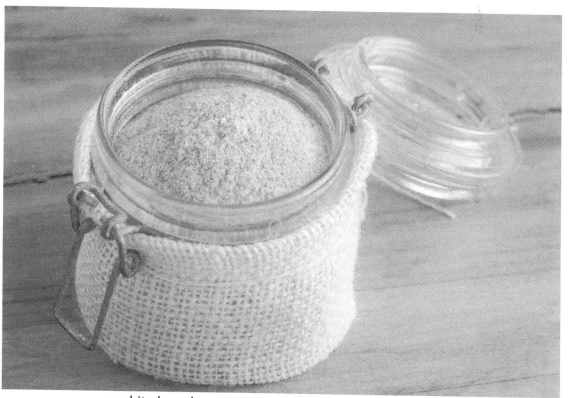

white bread.

Psyllium husk powder

- Psyllium husk powder – This powder is almost all fiber, so you'll want to add plenty of liquids in your baking, but in combination with other low-carb flours it can make your keto breads and muffins close in texture to their high-carb cousins.

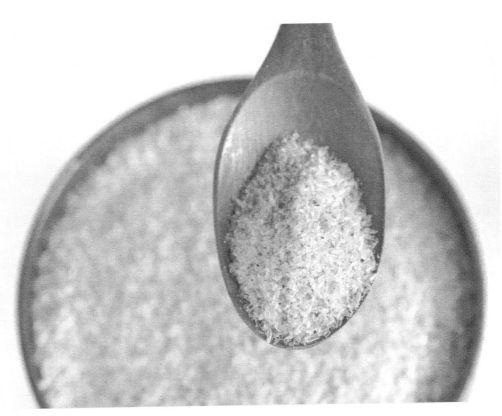

Spoonful of psyllium husks

- Psyllium husks – The whole husk is best used in doughs that need the stretchiness you would find in wheat flour. Breads, pizza dough, tortillas; the low-carb versions really benefit from the addition of psyllium husks.

- Flax meal – This can be used as a flour and also as an egg substitute. Just keep in mind that it will absorb plenty of liquid.

- Chia seeds – whole or ground, can be used to bread meats, added with other flavors. Chia seeds don't have much flavor on their own, so they won't compete with any spices you want to use.

- Pork rinds – when crumbled, work great as breading; they make a wonderful alternative to bread crumbs. Mix a little parmesan cheese with your pork rind crumbs and you've got a real taste treat breaded onto your fish or chicken.

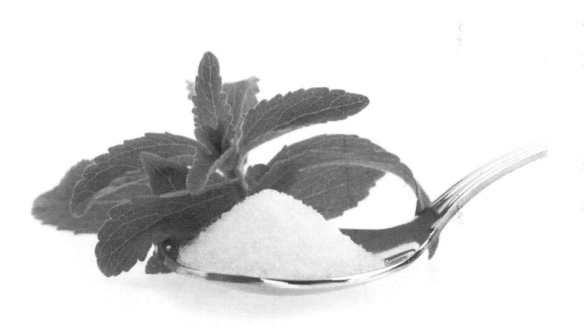

Sweetness Without The Sugar

Stevia plant with powdered extract

- Stevia – This plant-based source of sweetness can be found in powder or liquid form. It's calorie-free; technically it's so low-calorie that it qualifies to be called calorie-free. It's sweeter than sugar, so not as much is needed. Stevia won't caramelize like sugar, but it tastes great when used in any recipe that calls for sugar.

- Erythritol – Another natural sweetener. It isn't as sweet-tasting as sugar, so you may need to use a little more of it than you would of sugar, but it will satisfy your sweet tooth. It doesn't caramelize when heated, but otherwise it functions like sugar.

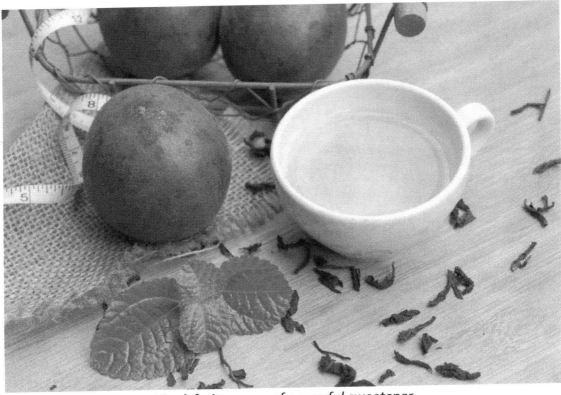
Monk fruit, source of powerful sweetener

- Monk fruit powder – The powdered form of this sweetener is 300 times as sweet as sugar, so a little will go a long way. It has a light flavor that makes it a perfect replacement for honey.

- Norbu – This product is a combination of monk fruit and erythritol. It caramelizes like "real" sugar.

- Swerve – A blend of erythritol, inulin, and various undefined flavors. Keep in mind that, while sugar-free, this sweetener does contain 5 grams of carbohydrates per teaspoon.

Sources of Fiber

One of the first things I discovered as I was researching the ketogenic diet was there are two types of fiber. Moreover, each one is necessary, for different reasons. Soluble fiber, as the name implies, dissolves in water. It comes in the form of gummy substances that glue to cholesterol and help flush it out of your body. Insoluble fiber, on the other hand, does not dissolve in water. Instead, it absorbs water, boosting your stool size, and speeding up the evacuation process.

The Scoop On Poop

Yes, I know it's a sensitive subject, but any discussion of dietary fiber will have to get around to it at some point. As your body is getting used to eating ketogenically, you may notice your digestive system is acting differently. This is most noticeable in the type and frequency of elimination of solid waste (read: poop). It's not uncommon to experience some fluctuation that ranges from mild constipation to diarrhea while you are establishing your new patterns of eating. Some of this can be stabilized by increasing your water intake.

People on the ketogenic diet generally report that their bowel movements are less frequent and the stool size and quantity is much smaller than before. It is perfectly normal to only have one to two bowel evacuations in a week's time. This means your body is processing your food more effectively; consequently there is much less waste to be dealt with.

If, however, you are continuing to experience either constipation and/or diarrhea, here's a rule of thumb that may help you. If you can't poop, increase your intake of insoluble fiber. If you can't stop pooping, however, you'll want to increase your amount of soluble fiber.

Most plants contain some of both kind of fiber. However, there are a few that major on one type or the other.

Sources Of Soluble Fiber (To Treat Diarrhea):

- Flax seeds

- Nuts

- Guar gum

- Psyllium

Sources Of Insoluble Fiber (To Treat Constipation):

- Avocado

- Chia seeds, ground – make a pudding by soaking in hot water or milk.

- Flax seeds, ground – mix with chia seeds and water or milk to make a pudding or by itself.

- An aside: constipation can be caused by ingesting too much dairy. Try cutting back on the dairy usage and see if the problem subsides.

Oils And Other Fats

- MCT oil – This oil provides medium chain triglycerides in much higher concentrations than you could ingest in natural food sources. MCTs are easily turned into ketones by your liver, making them a wonderful supplement for ketogenic dieters. You can find many uses for MCT oil. Use it in salad dressing or mayonnaise. Many people add it to their coffee for a morning pick-me-up. Try stirring a spoonful into your bowl of soup. You can add it to almost anything.

- Coconut oil – Boosts your immune system and helps your body digest food.

- Olive oil – The least processed of the oils, full of flavor and nutritional goodness. Should not be heated above 325 degrees Fahrenheit to avoid losing some of its nutritional properties.

- Avocado oil – Although not as common as olive or coconut oils, can be safely heated to above 400 degrees Fahrenheit.

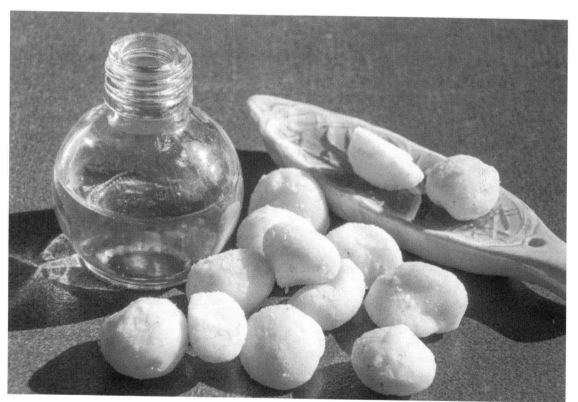

Macadamia Oil

- Macadamia oil – High smoke point, also mild in flavor, making it an excellent alternative to olive oil in mayonnaise.

- Flaxseed oil – Many of the same properties as the seed.

- Butter – Low smoke point, but oh, the flavor!

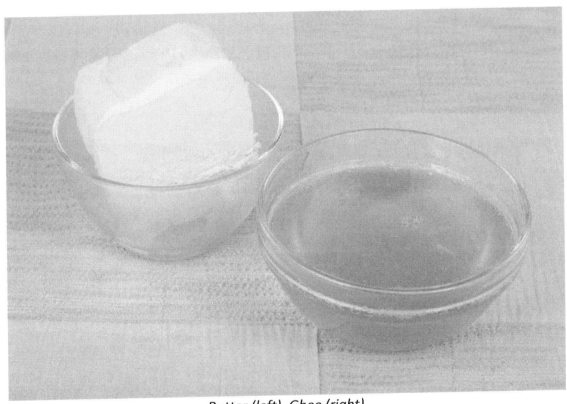

Butter (left), Ghee (right)

- Ghee – If you can't handle dairy, you just might be able to handle ghee! This clarified butter has all the casein and lactose removed in the process of getting rid of all the water and milk fats. This leaves you with an oil with a very high smoke point that has a slightly nutty buttery flavor. It is known to help establish a healthy digestive system, even as it effectively removes toxins.

- Don't forget the bacon grease! It adds great flavor to roasted vegetables, soup, you name it. And it makes a mouthwatering mayonnaise.

Other Atypical Ingredients

- Aioli – A combination of the French words for "oil" and "garlic", this tasty sauce can serve as a mayonnaise of sorts, as a dip, or a dollop can be served atop chicken to bring out the best of its flavors. You'll find a recipe in Chapter 10. A simple form of aioli can also be found in the recipe for Cauliflower Fish Cakes With Aioli, in Chapter 9.

- Cacao – healthier than the more intensively processed cocoa, but it still has a few carbohydrates to watch out for.

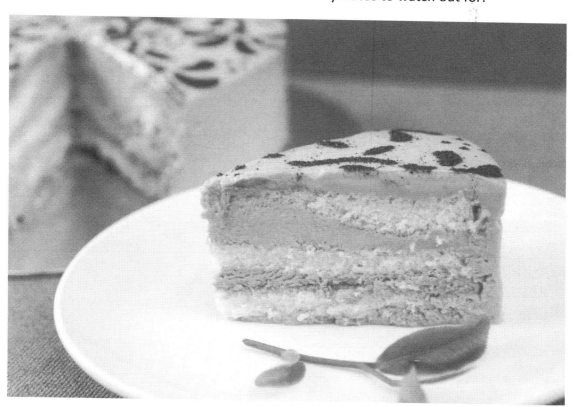

Matcha powder can be used for baking.

- Matcha Powder – comes from green tea but is healthier than the tea because it is made using the entire tea leaf. It's primarily used in smoothies, but creative souls are now using it for desserts as well.

Now that you have a better idea of the more unusual items you will encounter in ketogenic recipes, let's delve into the recipes themselves, starting off with some tasty appetizers.

Chapter 2: Delicious Appetizers

Appetizers are great to eat as snacks or for party time. When you are on the ketogenic diet and go to a party, it can be a challenge to find something you can eat. Now you can throw your own party with some of these appetizers. You can make regular tidbits for anybody not on the diet, but I warn you; your guests may well prefer the low-carb items. You'll probably want to hide some, just to ensure that you get a taste!

Apple And Ham Flatbread

Nutritional Information Per Serving Per Serving			
Yield:	8 servings	Serving Size:	1 piece
Calories:	255	Fat:	20 grams
Carbohydrates:	4 grams	Protein:	16 grams
Fiber:	10.3 grams		

Believe it or not, this flatbread crust is low-carb and delicious. It does *not* taste like cardboard! Combining it with ham and apples really makes a statement on your table. You can use the crust recipe for other things like pizza, as well. You'll want to slice the apples very thin, paper thin if you can, with a vegetable peeler. The ham should also be sliced thin and cut into strips. I use deli ham that I fold and slice myself.

You will need a double boiler for this recipe. If you don't have one, you can approximate one by using a saucepan with a mixing bowl that fits over the top, allowing the water to boil inside the saucepan and gently heat what is in the bowl.

Ingredients:

Crust:

- 2 cups part-skim Mozzarella cheese, grated

- 2 tablespoons cream cheese

- ¼ cup almond flour

- ½ teaspoon salt

- ⅛ teaspoon thyme

Topping:

- 1 cup part-skim Mozzarella cheese, grated

- ½ small red onion

- ½ small apple

- 4 ounces deli ham

- ⅛ teaspoon rosemary

- salt and pepper to taste

Directions:

1. Preheat the oven to 425 degrees Fahrenheit. Have ready a 12-inch pizza pan or a cookie sheet that will accommodate a 12-inch crust. Cut two pieces of parchment paper at least two inches larger than the pan or cookie sheet and set aside.

2. Pour water into the bottom of the double boiler and bring it to a boil. Into the top, drop in the two cups of Mozzarella cheese, the cream cheese, almond flour, salt, and thyme, giving it a quick mix with a fork.

3. Keep mixing with the fork; once the cheese starts to melt and it begins to look like everything will hold together, pour the mixture onto one piece of parchment. Carefully knead the dough so it becomes smooth and elastic, but be careful not to burn your fingers and hands. It will be hot.

4. Roll the dough into a ball and set it in the middle of the parchment paper. Pat this into a circle and lay the other piece of parchment over the top. Use a rolling pin to roll out into a 12-inch circle.

5. Slide the crust, including the bottom piece of parchment, onto the pizza pan. Prick it all over with the fork.

6. Set the crust inside the oven for six to eight minutes, until it's a rich golden brown. Do not over-bake. Take the crust out and set it aside. Lower the oven temperature to 350 degrees Fahrenheit.

7. While still hot, sprinkle a quarter cup of Mozzarella cheese over the top of the crust and let it cool.

8. Peel the red onion and cut half of it into very thin slices. Do not peel the apple, but core it and use only half of it. Use a vegetable peeler to make paper-thin slices. Tear the deli ham into one-inch pieces.

9. Arrange the onion slices on the crust and add the apple slices on top. Cover this with the ham pieces.

10. Sprinkle the rest of the cheese on top, and then scatter the entire pizza with thyme, salt, and pepper. Go easy on the salt if you are salt-sensitive. The ham may well be salty enough.

11. Bake for five to seven more minutes, until crust is golden brown. Take out of the oven and slide the flatbread, parchment and all, onto a cooling rack. Cool for three minutes, transfer to a cutting board and cut into eight pieces.

Baba Ganoush (Eggplant Dip)

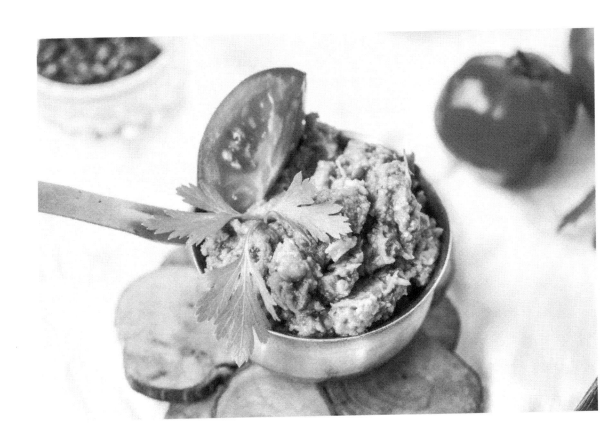

Nutritional Information Per Serving			
Yield:	varies	Serving Size:	⅓ cup
Calories:	110	Fat:	8 grams
Carbohydrates:	10 grams	Protein:	3 grams
Fiber:	5 grams		

Baba Ganoush

I love baba ganoush and the eggplant makes it perfect for the keto diet. This spicy flavorful mixture is used like a dip with raw veggies or on the sesame crackers you'll find a recipe for later on in this chapter.

Ingredients:

- 1 medium eggplant or two small ones

- 3 tablespoons lemon juice

36

- 2 cloves garlic (more, if you like garlic)

- ¼ cup tahini paste

- 1 teaspoon sea salt

- ½ teaspoon Hungarian paprika

- 2 to 3 tablespoons fresh parsley (do not use dried)

- Olive oil

Directions:

1. Set the oven to broil and preheat.

2. Prick the eggplant all over with a fork, then set it in a casserole dish that has been either lined with foil or coated with non-stick spray.

3. Set it under the broiler and leave it there until the skin begins to char. You will have to watch it carefully, as this happens quickly.

4. Flip over the eggplant so the other side starts to char. Poke a fork into the eggplant and if it isn't tender yet, reduce oven temp to 400 degrees and bake the eggplant about eight more minutes. The eggplant should be very soft inside.

5. Remove from the oven and let it cool.

6. Cut the eggplant in half and scoop out the inside, placing it in a blender or food processor. Do not use the charred skins; throw them away.

7. Add the lemon juice, peeled garlic cloves, Tahini paste, salt, paprika and fresh chopped parsley; blend until almost smooth.

8. Place the contents in a large bowl and drizzle a little olive oil on top. Sprinkle with a little more parsley for garnish. Serve with crackers or raw vegetables for dipping.

Buffalo Chicken Strips

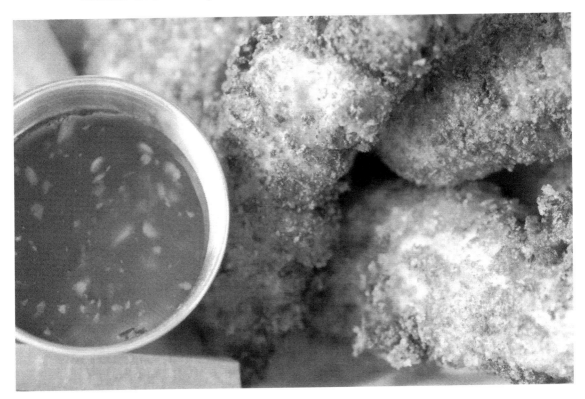

Nutritional Information Per Serving			
Yield:	3 servings	Serving Size:	3 strips
Calories:	683	Fat:	60 grams
Carbohydrates:	18 grams	Protein:	90 grams
Fiber:	9 grams		

Buffalo Chicken Strips

You absolutely cannot have an appetizer party without buffalo chicken in some form. This recipe for buffalo chicken strips is perfect for appetizers. You can also turn it into dinner, if you wish.

Ingredients:

- 1 tablespoon paprika
- 1 tablespoon chili powder
- 1 teaspoon salt
- 2 teaspoons pepper
- 1 teaspoon onion powder
- 1 teaspoon garlic powder
- 5 chicken breasts
- ¾ cup almond flour
- 4 tablespoons olive oil
- ½ cup hot sauce
- 3 tablespoons butter
- 3 tablespoons blue or feta cheese crumbles
- 2 eggs
- 1 teaspoon salt

Directions:

1. Preheat the oven to 400 degrees Fahrenheit.

2. In a small bowl, whisk together the paprika, chili powder, salt pepper, onion powder, and garlic powder. Set aside.

3. Pound out the chicken breasts to a half inch thick and cut them into two chunky halves.

4. Divide your spice mix into three equal portions.

5. Sprinkle one portion of the spice mix all over the chicken breasts, flip them over, and sprinkle the second portion of the spice mix on the other side.

6. In a bowl, mix the almond flour with the final portion of the spice mix. Use a whisk to combine well.

7. In another bowl, crack the eggs and whisk them thoroughly.

8. Dip a piece of chicken in the egg mixture, pull it out to let the excess drip off, then drop it in the almond flour mixture, making sure both sides are completely coated.

9. Place a cooling rack over a baking sheet covered with foil. Lay the chicken pieces on the rack. Bake for 15 minutes.

10. Remove from the oven and turn the broiler on. Drizzle two tablespoons of olive oil over the chicken. Broil for five minutes.

11. Flip the chicken over and drizzle with the rest of the olive oil. Broil again for five minutes, and remove from the oven.

12. Place the hot sauce and butter in a saucepan. Stir until the butter melts.

Serve the chicken with hot sauce slathered on top and cheese crumbled over it all.

Cheesy Spinach Puffs

Nutritional Information Per Serving			
Yield:	30 servings	Serving Size:	1 puff
Calories:	60	Fat:	5 grams

Carbohydrates:	0.8 grams	Protein:	2 grams
Fiber:	0 grams		

You won't have any leftover spinach puffs if you serve them at a party. I make these just to have snacks around the house, they are so good. The key is to get the spinach as dry as possible.

Ingredients:

- 1 16-ounce package frozen spinach

- 4 tablespoons salted butter

- 1 cup almond flour

- 2 eggs

- ⅓ cup feta cheese, crumbled

- ⅓ cup Parmesan cheese, grated

- 1 teaspoon salt

- ¼ teaspoon pepper

- 1 tablespoon onion powder

- 1 teaspoon garlic powder

- 3 tablespoons heavy whipping cream

Directions:

1. Prepare a cookie sheet by covering the surface with parchment paper.

2. Thaw the spinach completely and drain the liquid. Squeeze out as much moisture as you can.

3. Preheat the oven to 350 degrees Fahrenheit.

4. Place the drained spinach in a food processor and add the butter, almond flour, eggs, cheeses, salt, pepper, onion powder, garlic powder, and heavy whipping cream. Process until smooth.

5. Cover the mixture and chill it in the refrigerator for at least 15 minutes.

6. Shape the dough into one-inch balls and place them, separated, on the cookie sheet.

7. Bake for 12 minutes or until lightly brown. Cool on the cookie sheet.

8. Store in an airtight container.

Cheeseburger Muffins

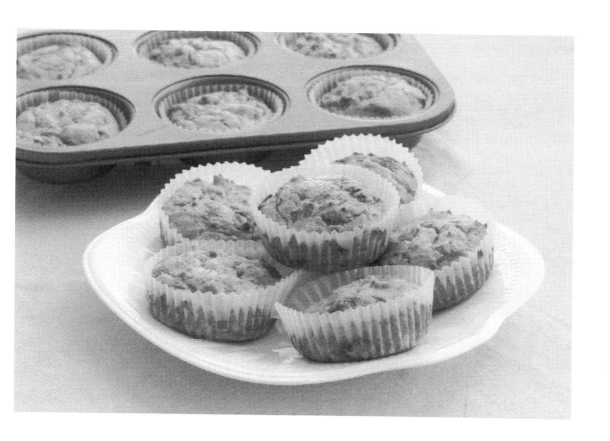

Nutritional Information Per Serving			
Yield:	9 servings	Serving Size:	1 muffin
Calories:	255	Fat:	20 grams
Carbohydrates:	5 grams	Protein:	15 grams
Fiber:	2 grams		

Cheeseburger Muffins

These little muffins are perfect for appetizers and they really do taste like cheeseburgers. They are made with flaxseed meal and almond flour to cut down on the carbs.

Ingredients:

Filling:

- 1 pound lean ground beef

- ½ teaspoon garlic powder

- ½ teaspoon onion powder

- 2 tablespoons tomato paste

- salt and pepper to taste

Buns:

- ½ cup flaxseed meal

- ½ cup almond flour

- 1 teaspoon baking powder

- ¼ teaspoon salt

- ¼ teaspoon pepper

- 2 eggs

- ¼ cup sour cream

Toppings:

- ½ cup shredded cheddar cheese

- dill pickle slices

- 2 tablespoons mustard

- 2 tablespoons low sugar ketchup

Directions:

1. Preheat the oven to 350 degrees Fahrenheit.

2. Place the ground beef in a skillet coated with non-stick spray, then sprinkle over it the garlic and onion powder.

Mix in well and brown the meat. Add the tomato paste, salt, and pepper and cook through. Remove from the heat and set aside.

3. In a bowl, combine the flaxseed meal, flour, baking powder, salt, and pepper. Whisk to combine.

4. In another bowl whisk the egg together with the sour cream.

5. Add the dry ingredients gradually to the egg mixture, beating well after each addition.

6. Divide the bun dough among nine muffin cups, lined with cupcake paper.

7. Indent the dough in the middle so it will rise up the sides of the cups. Leave some dough at the bottom of the cup. Fill the center with the ground beef mixture.

8. Bake for 15 to 20 minutes or until the muffins are lightly browned on the side.

9. Remove from the oven and top with the cheese. Set in the broiler for a couple minutes, just to melt the cheese.

10. Remove from muffin cups or tins.

11. Top with any or all of the toppings.

Cheesy Spinach Rolls With Apple-Slaw Topping

Nutritional Information Per Serving			
Yield:	3 servings	Serving Size:	5 rolls
Calories:	670	Fat:	67 grams
Carbohydrates:	20 grams	Protein:	32 grams
Fiber:	4		

These rolls are perfect for breakfast or lunch. The crust is made using both almond and coconut flour, making it a flavorful low-carb treat that is well complemented by the topping. I prefer to use a tart apple, such as Granny Smith, for the slaw. The slaw is tasty enough that I often expand the recipe and use it alongside other dishes.

Ingredients:

Crust:

- 2½ cups part-skim Mozzarella cheese

- 6 tablespoons coconut flour

- ½ cup almond flour

- 2 eggs

- ¼ teaspoon sea salt

Filling:

- 1 teaspoon olive oil

- 6 ounces fresh spinach

- ¼ cup Parmesan

- 4 ounces cream cheese

- ⅛ teaspoon sea salt

Topping:

- ¾ cup of packaged coleslaw salad mix

- 1 apple

- ¼ cup mayonnaise

- ⅛ teaspoon sea salt

Directions:

1. Preheat the oven to 350 degrees Fahrenheit.

2. In a skillet, add the olive oil and sauté the spinach leaves until they wilt.

3. Add the shredded Parmesan and the cream cheese, stirring constantly until everything melts and the spinach is thoroughly coated. Remove from heat and set aside.

4. Make the crust by placing the Mozzarella cheese in the microwave on high for about 30 seconds and then in 10 second intervals until the cheese is soft and pliable.

5. Add the coconut and almond flours and mix well with a fork. Add the eggs and salt and mix thoroughly together. Knead as necessary to persuade the crust to stick together.

6. Place the dough in the center of one piece of parchment paper and cover with another sheet. Flatten the dough with a rolling pin until the resulting circle is an eighth of an inch thick.

7. Use a pizza cutter to slice into three by four-inch triangles.

8. Spoon a half teaspoon of the filling onto the tip half of the triangle and carefully roll it toward the broad base. Place the rolls on a parchment-covered cookie sheet that has been coated with non-stick spray.

9. Bake for 18 minutes or until the crust becomes a light golden brown. Let it cool for 10 minutes.

10. Make the slaw by placing the coleslaw mix in a bowl. Peel and core the apple. Grate it into the slaw mix. Add the mayonnaise and salt and mix well. Place in the refrigerator until ready to serve.

11. To serve, place a dollop of the slaw on top of each roll.

Ground Chicken Meatballs With Kick

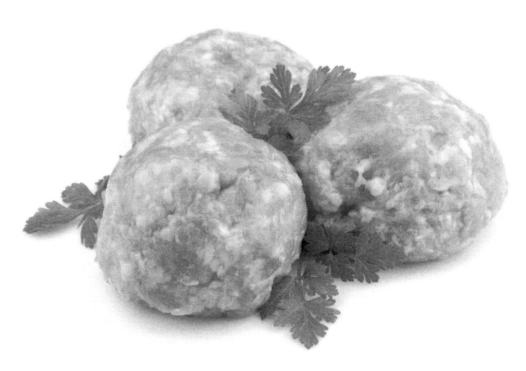

Chicken meatballs, before cooking

Nutritional Information Per Serving			
Yield:	4 servings	Serving Size:	4 meatballs
Calories:	368	Fat:	26 grams
Carbohydrates:	2 grams	Protein:	31 grams
Fiber:	1 gram		

Ground Chicken Meatballs

I stick toothpicks into these meatball flavor blasts for easy access. The kick comes from the jalapeno pepper hidden deep inside.

Instead of high-carb breadcrumbs for the extender, you'll find crushed pork rinds.

Ingredients:

- 2 tablespoons ground pork rinds

- ¼ cup onion, finely diced

- 1-pound ground chicken (If you can find ground dark meat, all the better.)

- 1 small jalapeno, seeded and diced finely

- 4 ounces cream cheese, softened

- ¼ cup cheddar cheese, shredded

- salt and pepper to taste

Directions:

1. Mix the ground pork rinds with the diced onions in a bowl, along with the salt and pepper.

2. Add the ground chicken and egg. Mix with your hands until the ingredients are well combined. Place in the refrigerator to chill for 15 to 20 minutes.

3. Preheat the oven to 350 degrees Fahrenheit.

4. Mix the jalapeno, cream cheese, and cheddar cheese in a small bowl and set aside.

5. Remove the chicken mixture from the refrigerator.

6. Scoop out a little of the chicken mixture into your palm, flatten it and make an indentation in the center. Place about a teaspoon of the jalapeno/cheese mixture into the

center of the meat and form the meatball around it. The completed meatballs should be no larger than golf balls.

7. Place the meatballs in a non-stick sprayed baking dish and bake for 30 minutes, until chicken is cooked and brown on the bottom.

8. Transfer to serving dish, add toothpicks, and enjoy.

Low-Carb Sesame Crackers

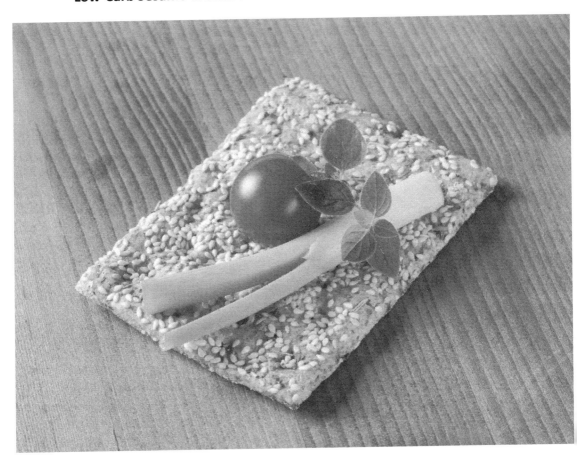

Nutritional Information Per Serving			
Yield:	4 servings	Serving Size:	10 crackers
Calories:	197	Fat:	17 grams

Carbohydrates:	6 grams	Protein:	8 grams
Fiber	2 grams		

Sesame Crackers

These little crackers are great to dip into almost anything, or just to eat by themselves. They are made with naturally low-carbohydrate almond flour and the sesame seeds, which enhance the flavor.

Ingredients:

- 3 tablespoons sesame seeds

- ¼ teaspoon baking soda

- 1 cup almond flour

- ¼ teaspoon salt

- ¼ teaspoon pepper

- 1 egg

- Additional salt and pepper to taste

Directions:

1. Move the oven rack to the middle of the oven and preheat to 350 degrees Fahrenheit.

2. In a large bowl mix the sesame seeds, baking soda, almond flour, salt, and pepper.

3. Beat the egg well. Gradually add the dry ingredients until it is all worked in and a dough forms. Divide the dough in half.

4. Put a large sheet of parchment paper on the counter and coat with non-stick spray. Set one half of the dough in the

center of the parchment paper. Cover with a second sheet of parchment paper that has been similarly treated.

5. Using a rolling pin, flatten the dough into a sixteenth of an inch thick rectangle.

6. Remove the top sheet of parchment paper and use a pizza cutter to slice the dough into 20 squares, but do not separate them. Sprinkle with a little salt and pepper. Slide parchment paper and all onto a cookie sheet.

7. Bake for 15 to 20 minutes or until lightly browned. Let it cool for a bit before moving onto a cooling rack. Once cool, break them into individual crackers.

8. Repeat this process with the second half of dough.

9. Store in an airtight container.

Scotch Eggs

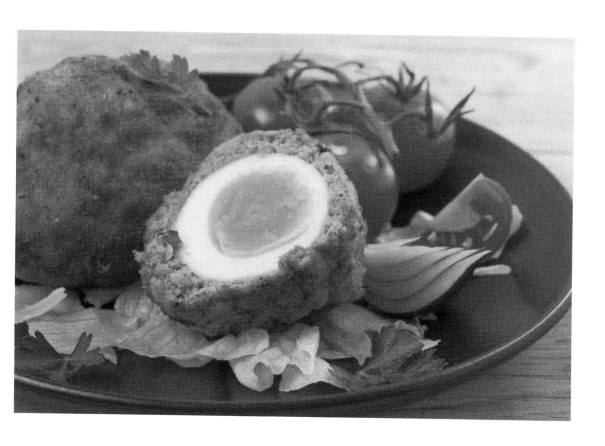

Nutritional Information Per Serving			
Yield:	6 servings	Serving Size:	1 egg
Calories:	300	Fat:	21 grams
Carbohydrates:	16 grams	Protein:	12 grams
Fiber	0 grams		

Scotch Eggs

This recipe is a little unusual, especially when you consider that you bury them in meat. The eggs are hard boiled and I like them to be a little firm, although many people prefer them slightly soft. To boil the eggs, just cover them in a saucepan with cold water and bring to a boil. For a firm egg boil five to seven minutes and for a softer egg, go three to four minutes. I do not suggest you go more than the seven minutes because you also bake the eggs and they will cook further and firm up even more. We used to find these at Renaissance Fairs and they are good for keeping you from getting hungry.

Ingredients:

- 6 eggs

- 1 pound ground Italian sausage (avoid sausage with high sugar content)

- ¼ teaspoon sage

- ¼ teaspoon parsley

- ¼ teaspoon rosemary

- ½ teaspoon salt

Directions:

1. Soft boil the eggs by placing them in a saucepan, covering them with cold water, and bringing it to a boil. Let the water boil for three to four minutes. You want to boil them as soft as possible, because you will also be baking them. When your eggs are cooked to your liking, let them cool, then peel and set them aside.

2. Preheat the oven to 350 degrees Fahrenheit and prepare a 9 by 13-inch casserole dish with non-stick spray.

3. Place the ground sausage in a bowl with the spices. Mix thoroughly.

4. Take a handful of pork and shape it into a thin, flat patty. Place the boiled egg in the center and gently shape the meat around the egg, encasing it entirely.

5. Set the covered eggs in the baking dish and bake for 30 minutes.

Spicy Smoky Hot Crab Dip

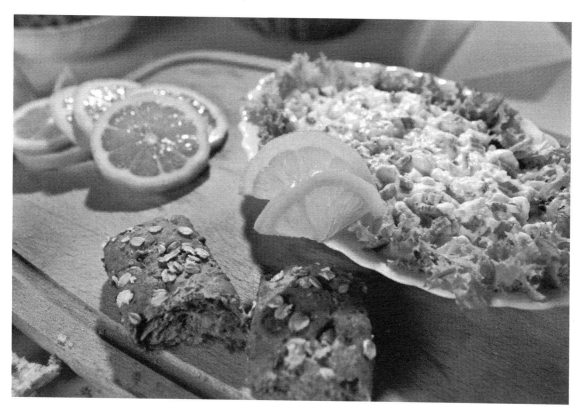

Nutritional Information Per Serving			
Yield:	20 servings	Serving Size:	¼ cup
Calories:	125	Fat:	8 grams
Carbohydrates:	2 grams	Protein:	11 grams
Fiber	0 grams		

Crab Dip

This dip is simply delicious. You can use either lump crab or claw meat and it only takes about half an hour to make.

Ingredients:

- 16 strips bacon

- 16 ounces cream cheese, softened

- 1 cup sour cream

- 1 cup mayonnaise

- 3 poblano peppers

- 8 green onions

- 7 cloves of garlic

- 3½ tablespoons lemon juice

- 2 cups Parmesan cheese, divided

- 2 12-ounce cans of crab meat

- Fresh cracked pepper to taste

Directions:

1. Preheat your oven to 350 degrees Fahrenheit.

2. Cut the bacon into small pieces. Heat a large sauté pan on medium and fry the bacon until the pieces are brown and crisp. Drain the fat and drain on a paper towel.

3. Add the cream cheese, the sour cream, and the mayonnaise. Mix well; a few lumps are allowed, though.

4. Clean and dice the peppers, mince the onions (reserving about two tablespoons for garnish), and peel and mince the garlic. Combine them in a bowl with the lemon juice and one cup of grated Parmesan cheese. Add to the sour cream mixture and stir to combine.

5. Add the crab meat and pepper and fold it gently into the mixture with a rubber spatula. Only break up the crab meat enough to disperse it through the dip.

6. Scrape into an oven-safe dish treated with non-stick spray. Spread it evenly and top with the rest of the Parmesan cheese.

7. Bake for 20 minutes or until golden brown and bubbly.

8. Garnish with some of the onions and serve with raw veggies or ketogenic crackers.

Chapter 3: Scrumptious Salads and Dressings

I enjoy a salad for lunch because it is light and refreshing. Yes, you can eat salads as part of the ketogenic diet; you'll just need to balance out any carbohydrates that sneak in, with offsetting protein and fats throughout the day. The following salads contain enough protein and fats to serve as meals. I have also included some yummy salad dressings that can be used on any salad, even a small side salad.

Cauliflower "Potato" Salad

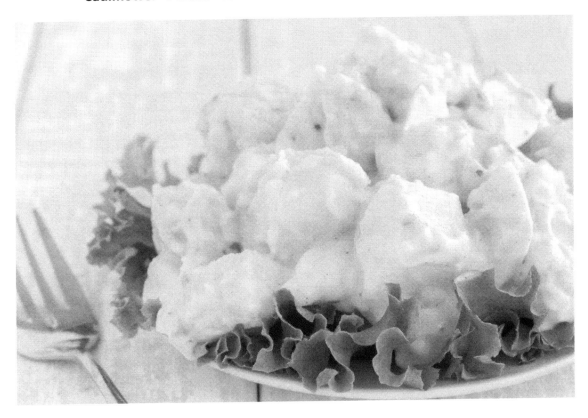

Nutritional Information Per Serving			
Yield:	8 servings	Serving Size:	½ cup
Calories:	169	Fat:	15 grams

Carbohydrates:	5 grams	Protein:	5 grams
Fiber	2 grams		

Cauliflower Potato Salad

I love potato salad and, as you know, potatoes have too many carbs to be eaten on a keto diet. This tasty alternative does have a different flavor, but it is just as delicious and heart-warming as potato salad. Cauliflower is one of the lowest carbohydrate vegetables you can find. You can use it as a main dish or as a hearty side. The nutritional values here are for a side dish, so adjust accordingly if you are using it as a main course.

Ingredients:

- 3 eggs, hard boiled

- 4 strips bacon

- 1 medium head of cauliflower

- ¼ cup red onion, chopped

- 2 stalks celery, chopped finely

- 3 tablespoons chives, diced

- ½ tablespoon yellow mustard

- ½ cup mayonnaise

- ½ tablespoon apple cider vinegar

- ½ teaspoon salt

- ¼ teaspoon black pepper

Directions:

1. Peel and chop the eggs.

2. Fry the bacon until crisp. Cool, then break into small pieces.

3. Chop the cauliflower into bite-sized pieces and put in a microwave safe bowl. Dampen a paper towel and place it over the top of the bowl. Microwave on high for about three minutes. Remove the paper towel and dampen it again. Cover the bowl and microwave for another three minutes, or until the cauliflower pieces are tender; then set aside to cool.

4. Combine the celery, onion, and chives in a large bowl.

5. Add the cooled cauliflower, chopped eggs, and bacon to the bowl.

6. In another bowl, whisk together the mustard, mayonnaise, and vinegar. Add the salt and pepper and whisk to combine.

7. Add the mustard mixture to the cauliflower mixture and fold in with a rubber spatula until everything is coated. Put in the refrigerator to cool for at least three hours before eating.

Fresh Chicken Salad

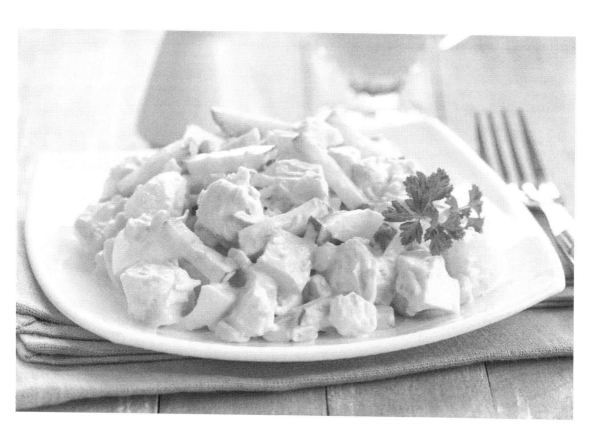

Nutritional Information Per Serving			
Yield:	4 servings	Serving Size:	½ cup
Calories:	367	Fat:	25 grams
Carbohydrates:	2 grams	Protein:	34 grams
Fiber	0.25 grams		

Fresh Chicken Salad

This chicken salad tastes very fresh because of the lemon juice and sour cream it contains. The included pecans also add a fresh crunch. You can serve this salad inside a hollowed-out tomato or over some lettuce leaves. You can use leftover chicken meat or you can bake or boil chicken thighs and break up the meat. You can also use canned chicken if you prefer, but it's not my favorite. Note: if you aren't using thigh meat, your nutritional values may be a little different.

Ingredients:

- 1½ pounds boneless, skinless chicken thighs

- 1 tablespoon coconut oil

- 2 tablespoons sour cream

- ⅓ cup mayonnaise

- ½ lemon, juiced

- 2 stalks of celery

- 1½ tablespoons parsley

- 1½ tablespoons chives

- ¼ teaspoon salt

- ⅛ teaspoon pepper

- ¼ cup pecans

Directions:

1. Cut the chicken meat into bite-sized pieces. Place the coconut oil in a skillet and add the chicken pieces. Cook the chicken. Let cool completely.

2. In a small bowl, whisk together the sour cream, mayonnaise, and lemon juice. Set aside.

3. Chop the celery, parsley, chives, salt, and pepper and place in a large bowl. Add the sour cream mixture to the cooled chicken and mix thoroughly. Add the pecans and toss to combine.

Greek Lemon Dressing

Nutritional Information Per Serving			
Yield:	8 servings	Serving Size:	2 tablespoons
Calories:	82	Fat:	8 grams
Carbohydrates:	0.2 gram	Protein:	0 grams
Fiber	0.1 gram		

This dressing tastes very fresh over a green salad, but don't limit it to salad. A drizzle can also enhance cooked vegetables or fish dishes. I put all my ingredients in a glass jar, tighten down the lid, and shake to mix it. The jar stores it perfectly in the refrigerator. When I want to use it, I just shake and pour.

Ingredients:

- ¼ cup lemon juice, fresh squeezed

- ¼ teaspoon salt

- Pinch of black pepper

- 2 teaspoons Greek oregano

- 1 teaspoon Dijon mustard

- 2 cloves garlic, peeled and minced fine

- ¾ cup extra virgin olive oil

Directions:

1. Put all ingredients except the olive oil in the jar, screw the lid down tight, and shake well.

2. Add the olive oil. Shake well until everything is combined and the mixture appears creamy.

3. Taste the mixture and adjust to taste. If it's too tart, add more olive oil. You can also adjust the salt or pepper to suit your preference.

Lemon-Avocado Tuna Salad

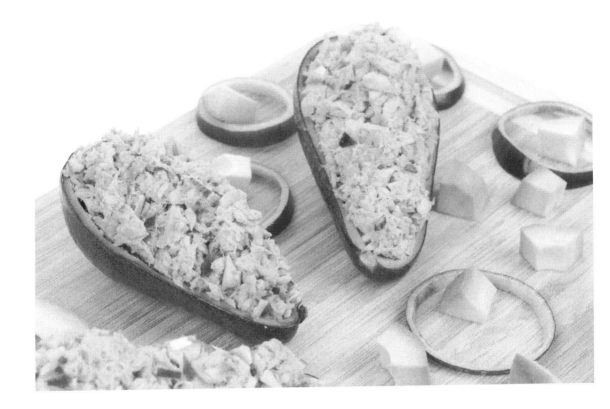

Nutritional Information Per Serving			
Yield:	2 servings	Serving Size:	½ total
Calories:	480	Fat:	40 grams
Carbohydrates:	11 grams	Protein:	45 grams
Fiber	8 grams		

Lemon-Avocado Tuna Salad

Tuna salad is a staple at our house. This one is a little different because of the lemon, which adds sunny freshness to balance the punch from the pepper. Oh, and don't forget the avocado, which adds the smoothness of comfort food to almost anything.

Ingredients:

- 1 teaspoon lemon juice
- ½ small avocado
- ⅓ cucumber
- 1 4.6-ounce can tuna
- 1 tablespoon mayonnaise
- 1 tablespoon mustard
- Salt and pepper to taste
- Lettuce leaves

Directions:

1. Squeeze the lemon juice from a lemon into a large bowl. Dice the avocado in small pieces and add to the bowl. Peel and dice the cucumber and add to the bowl. Combine the three ingredients well.

2. In another bowl, flake the tuna and mix with the mayonnaise and the mustard. Sprinkle with salt and pepper and mix.

3. Add the tuna combination to the lemon juice mixture and mix well.

4. Serve atop a lettuce leaf.

Low-Carb Creamy Ranch Dressing

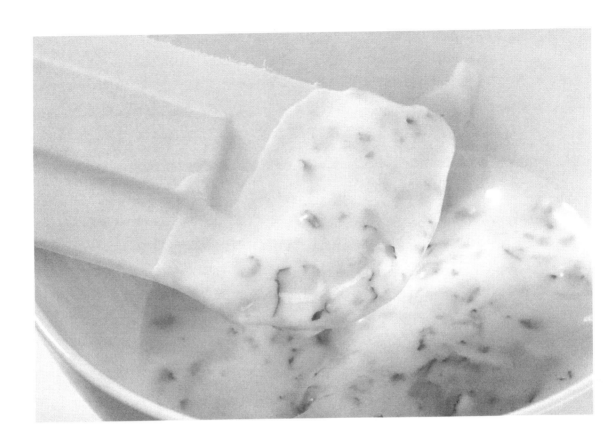

Nutritional Information Per Serving			
Yield:	24 servings	Serving Size:	1 tablespoon
Calories:	106	Fat:	11 grams
Carbohydrates:	0.6 grams	Protein:	0.65 grams
Fiber	0.08 grams		

Low-Carb Creamy Ranch Dressing

Ranch dressing is one of those staples in our house. We use it for more than salads. We dip raw vegetables in it for a snack. I dip chicken in it and slather it on top of other meats as well. This recipe calls for dried herbs instead of fresh ones; this avoids adding too much moisture to the mix and it adds a little more intensity to the flavor.

Ingredients:

- ½ cup sour cream

- 1 cup mayonnaise (optional: use the recipe in Chapter 10)

- ¼ cup heavy whipping cream

- ¼ teaspoon dill

- 2 tablespoons parsley

- ¼ teaspoon basil

- ¼ teaspoon garlic powder

- ¼ teaspoon onion powder

- ¼ teaspoon salt

- ¼ teaspoon pepper

Directions:

1. Put all the ingredients into a blender and blend for about 60 seconds.

2. Pour into a glass jar with a lid and store it in the refrigerator for several hours before serving.

3. The dressing will keep for about two months in the refrigerator.

Strawberry Vinaigrette Dressing

Nutritional Information Per Serving			
Yield:	8 servings	Serving Size:	2 Tbsp.
Calories:	113	Fat:	13 grams
Carbohydrates:	0.9 grams	Protein:	0.1 grams
Fiber	0.2 grams		

This dressing is low-carbohydrate and you can use it with all types of green salads. The best thing about it is, you can switch out the strawberries for raspberries or any other kind of fruit, if you feel adventurous. You can also make a grilled chicken salad and top it with this dressing.

Store your dressing in the refrigerator and it will keep for two to three weeks.

Ingredients:

- ½ cup strawberries, hulled and sliced

- 2 tablespoons balsamic vinegar

- ½ teaspoon dry mustard

- Stevia to taste, optional

- ½ cup extra virgin olive oil

Directions:

1. Place the strawberries in a blender or food processor and puree.

2. Add the vinegar and dry mustard. Add sweetener to taste and some optional salt if preferred.

3. Puree the olive oil into the mixture gradually, and serve.

Tamari Steak Salad

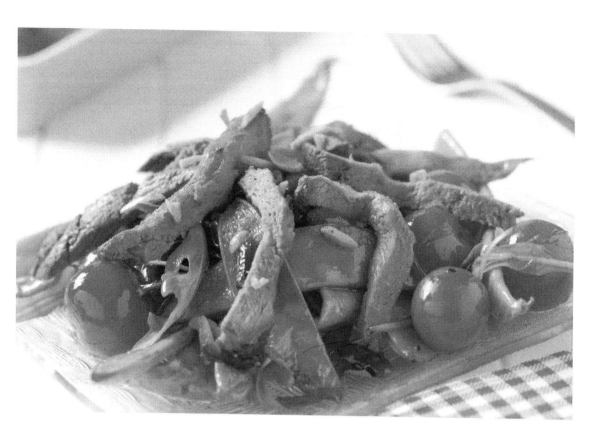

Nutritional Information Per Serving			
Yield:	2 servings	Serving Size:	½ total
Calories:	500	Fat:	37 grams
Carbohydrates:	4 grams	Protein:	33 grams
Fiber	2 grams		

Tamari Steak Salad

I love a good steak salad, and this is my "go to" recipe. You do have to plan ahead a little because the steak needs to marinate in the tamari sauce overnight, but it comes out very tender and delicious. You can grill or pan fry the steak. Top with the ranch dressing you'll find in this chapter, for a full-flavored meal.

Ingredients:

- 1 ½-pound steak

- ¼ cup tamari sauce

- 2.5 ounces salad greens

- 8 cherry tomatoes

- ½ red bell pepper

- 4 radishes

- ½ tablespoon lemon juice

- 1 tablespoon olive oil

- Olive oil

- Salt and pepper to taste

Directions:

1. Place the steak in a large re-closable plastic bag along with the Tamari sauce, close it, and stash in the refrigerator to marinate overnight.

2. Place the salad greens in a large bowl.

3. Clean the bell pepper and cut into slices, cut the cherry tomatoes in half, and slice the radishes thinly.

4. Place the sliced peppers, tomatoes, and radishes in the bowl, along with the salad greens.

5. In a small bowl whisk together the olive oil and lemon juice. Pour over the salad greens and toss to coat. Divide into the two serving bowls.

6. Pour a little olive oil in a frying pan and heat. Remove the steak from the marinade and place in the frying pan, seasoning it with salt and pepper. Cook on both sides to the desired amount of doneness.

7. Place the steak on a plate and let it set for one minute before slicing. Arrange one half of the slices on top of each bowl of greens and serve while warm.

Turkey Arugula Salad

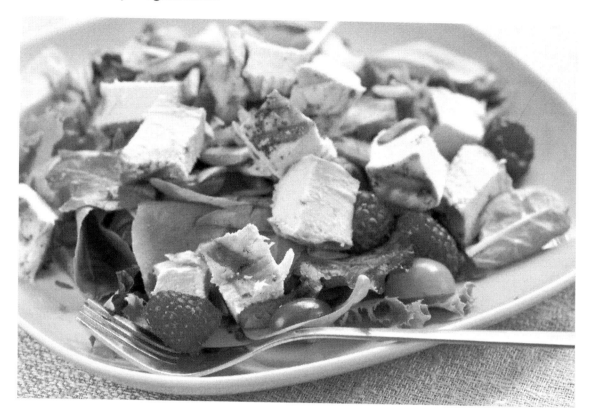

Nutritional Information Per Serving			
Yield:	2 servings	Serving Size:	½ total
Calories:	260	Fat:	15 grams
Carbohydrates:	9 grams	Protein:	20 grams
Fiber	3 grams		

turkey arugula salad

Use turkey cut from the breast or deli turkey for this recipe. I prefer turkey that I have cooked and cut from the breast.

This dish is very easy to make; you just toss everything together in a large bowl and serve it up. This recipe will provide you with two healthy-sized servings.

Ingredients:

- 4 ounces turkey breast

- 4 ounces arugula

- 1 cucumber

- 10 raspberries

- 2 tablespoons olive oil

- Juice from ½ lime

Directions:

1. Slice the turkey thinly and place in a large bowl.

2. Tear the arugula into bite-sized pieces and add to the turkey meat.

3. Peel and slice the cucumber and add to the bowl.

4. Toss in the raspberries.

5. In a small bowl, combine the olive oil with the lime juice and pour over the contents of the bowl.

6. Toss to combine and serve.

Zesty Low-Carb Italian Dressing

Nutritional Information Per Serving			
Yield:	16 servings	Serving Size:	½ ounce
Calories:	83	Fat:	9 grams
Carbohydrates:	0.54 grams	Protein:	0.11 grams

Fiber	0.16 grams	

This dressing will wake up your taste buds and make them happy. Use it on green salads or as a marinade for chicken, fish, or pork.

Ingredients:

- ¼ cup red wine vinegar

- 1 teaspoon lemon juice

- ⅔ cup olive oil

- 1 teaspoon fresh garlic, minced

- 1 teaspoon dry oregano

- 1 teaspoon dry rosemary

- 1 teaspoon dry basil

- ½ teaspoon salt

- ¼ teaspoon red pepper flakes

Directions:

1. Pour all the ingredients into the blender and blend for 30 to 40 seconds.

2. Pour into a glass jar and refrigerate at least three hours before serving.

3. Shake before using.

4. The dressing will last about one month in the refrigerator.

Zesty Taco Salad

Nutritional Information Per Serving			
Yield:	2 servings	Serving Size:	½ total
Calories:	521	Fat:	40 grams
Carbohydrates:	12 grams	Protein:	31 grams
Fiber	5 grams		

If you are on a ketogenic diet, you can't really have beans because of all the carbs, nor can you eat taco chips. Instead, use crisp bell peppers to give you the chips' crunch, and the avocado to add some of the texture beans would usually provide. This is another salad that tastes great with ranch dressing.

Ingredients:

- ½ pound ground beef

- 2 tablespoons taco seasoning

- 1 green onion

- ¼ cup bell pepper (I like red, but you can use any color you want)

- 2 tablespoons avocado, diced

- 2 tablespoons tomato, diced

- ½ small jalapeno, thin sliced (optional)

- 1 tablespoon chipotles in adobo sauce

- 4 cups romaine lettuce

- ½ cup cilantro

- ¼ cup cheddar cheese, shredded

- 4 tablespoons ranch dressing (also found in this chapter)

Directions:

1. Heat the ground beef with the taco seasoning in a skillet over medium heat. Stir and break up clumps with a wooden spoon. Cook all the way through and set aside.

2. Chop the onions and bell peppers and dice the avocado and tomato. Slice the jalapeno and chop the chipotle in adobe. Tear the lettuce into bite-sized pieces and chop the cilantro.

3. Place half of the lettuce and cilantro in one bowl and the other half in another bowl. Add the onion, bell pepper, tomato, and jalapenos to both bowls. Add the chipotle in adobo sauce and sprinkle cheddar cheese over top. Finish with the ranch dressing and serve.

Chapter 4: Tasty Soups and Stews

Soup was always a comfort food when I was growing up. A nice warm bowl not only warmed the body, but it also infused the soul with hope. You knew you were loved because someone took the time to make it for you. Soups and stews were always a great way to stretch a small piece of meat, back then.

The following soups and stews are low-carb versions of what you probably grew up on. No wimpy canned soup for you! These energizing stews use fresh ingredients for the heartiest flavors and the most complete nutrition.

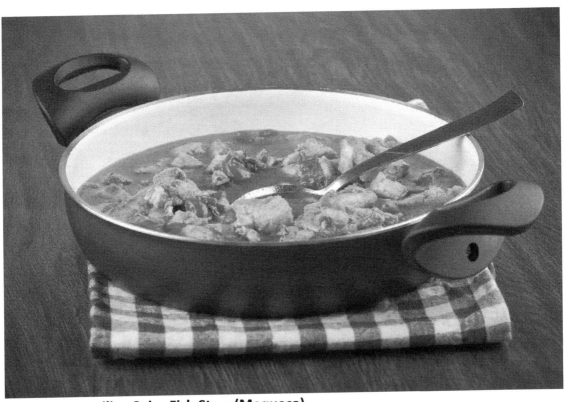

Brazilian Spicy Fish Stew (Moqueca)

Nutritional Information Per Serving			
Yield:	4 servings	Serving Size:	1 bowl
Calories:	428	Fat:	25 grams
Carbohydrates:	9 grams	Protein:	19 grams
Fiber	0 grams		

Moqueca

A friend from Brazil made this stew for me; it was so good I decided to include the recipe for you to enjoy. It is naturally low-carb and delicious.

Ingredients:

- 1 2-pound cod or whitefish, cut into bite-sized pieces

- 4 tablespoons fresh lime juice

- 2 tablespoons olive oil

- 1 jalapeños, seeded and chopped

- 1 onion, peeled and chopped

- 1 red bell pepper, chopped

- 1 yellow bell pepper, chopped

- 3 cloves garlic, peeled and chopped

- 2 teaspoons paprika

- 4 cups chicken bone broth

- 4 cups crushed tomatoes

- 1½ teaspoon sea salt

- ½ teaspoon black pepper

- 2 13.5-ounce cans light coconut milk

Directions:

1. Put the fish pieces in a glass bowl and add the lime juice and salt. Toss well and set aside to marinate while preparing everything else.

2. Heat the olive oil in a heavy, large pan and add the jalapeños, onion, and bell peppers. Sauté for about three minutes, until the onion is translucent.

3. Add the garlic and sauté for another 30 seconds.

4. Add the paprika, tomatoes, salt, and pepper and bring to a boil.

5. Add the fish with its marinade and stir. Put a lid on the pan and turn down the heat to low. Simmer about 10 minutes or until the fish will flake with a fork.

6. Serve with wedges of lime.

Chicken Zucchini-Noodle Soup

Nutritional Information Per Serving			
Yield:	2 servings	Serving Size:	1 bowl
Calories:	310	Fat:	10 grams
Carbohydrates:	6 grams	Protein:	34 grams
Fiber	2 grams		

If you *really* want noodles with your chicken soup, I found a recipe that gives you that satisfaction, but the noodles are made from thin ribbons of zucchini.

Ingredients:

- 1 deboned, skinless chicken breast, chopped into bite-sized pieces

- 1 tablespoon olive oil

- 3 cups chicken broth

- 1 green onion, chopped

- 1 stalk of celery, chopped

- 1 carrot, peeled and chopped

- 1 teaspoon chopped garlic

- 1 zucchini, peeled

- ¼ cup cilantro, chopped fine

- ¼ teaspoon salt

- ¼ teaspoon pepper

Directions:

1. Pound the chicken breast as flat as possible and chop the breast into bite-sized pieces.

2. Put the olive oil in a Dutch oven and sauté the chicken pieces until they are cooked through.

3. Add the broth and lower the heat to a simmer.

4. Add the onion, celery, carrot, and garlic and simmer for 15 minutes.

5. Meanwhile, use a potato peeler and run it down the length of the zucchini, to cut it into zucchini ribbons.

6. Add the ribbons, cilantro, salt, and pepper to the pot and simmer for 10 more minutes.

7. Serve hot.

Comforting Chicken Crock-Pot Stew

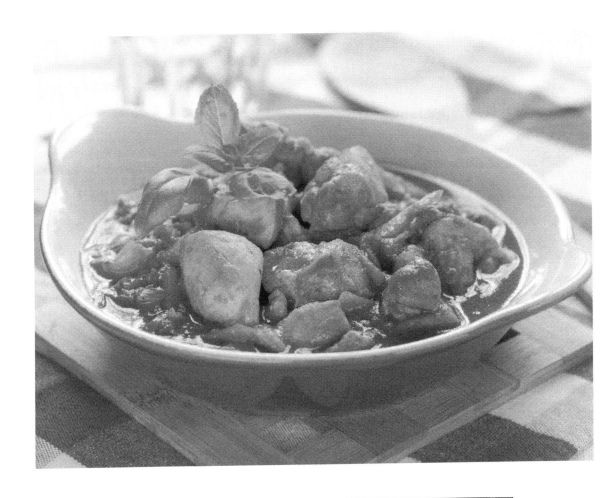

Nutritional Information Per Serving			
Yield:	4 servings	Serving Size:	1 cup
Calories:	228	Fat:	11 grams
Carbohydrates:	6 grams	Protein:	6 grams
Fiber	0 grams		

Chicken Crock-Pot Stew

This recipe yields a creamy stew that is thickened with xanthan gum. It is a little richer than you may be accustomed to, because it includes heavy cream. The use of fresh spinach adds hearty flavor to the pot.

Ingredients:

- 4 tablespoons olive oil, divided

- 2 cloves garlic, peeled and minced

- ½ cup onion, diced

- ½ cup carrots, diced

- ½ teaspoon salt

- ¼ teaspoon pepper

- 1 cup celery, diced

- 28 ounces chicken thighs, deboned, skin removed, and cut into one-inch pieces

- 2 cups chicken stock

- ¼ teaspoon dried thyme

- ½ teaspoon dried rosemary

- ½ teaspoon dried oregano

- 1 cup fresh spinach leaves

- ½ cup heavy cream

- ¼ to ½ teaspoon xanthan gum

Directions:

1. Heat a large skillet over medium high temperature and add two tablespoons of olive oil. Sauté the garlic and onion over medium heat for about three minutes or until the onion becomes tender. Add the carrots and sauté for three more minutes.

2. Pour the vegetables into a Crock-Pot that has been coated with non-stick spray.

3. Add the additional olive oil to the skillet. Salt and pepper the chicken thigh pieces and brown on all sides. Do not cook through.

4. Place in the bottom of the Crock-Pot.

5. Add the chicken stock, thyme, rosemary, and oregano. Cook on low for four hours or on the high setting for two hours.

6. Add the spinach and stir.

7. Add the heavy cream and turn the temperature setting to high.

8. Add a quarter teaspoon of xanthan gum at first and whisk occasionally while heating for 10 minutes. The mixture should thicken. If not, add a little more of the thickener and cook, whisking occasionally for another 10 minutes.

9. Serve while hot.

Economical Hamburger Veggie Soup

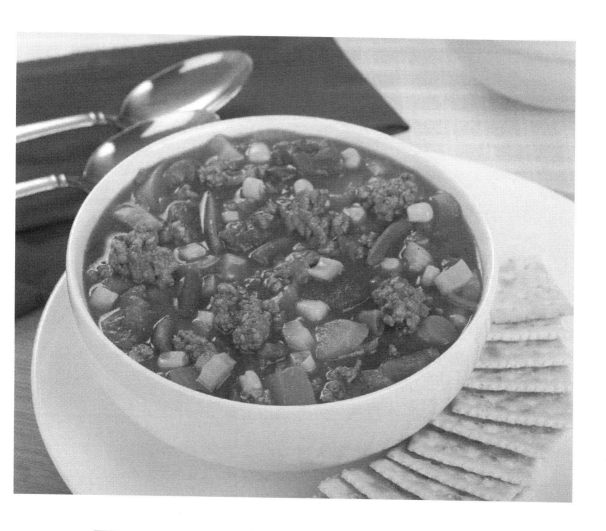

Nutritional Information Per Serving			
Yield:	10 servings	Serving Size:	1 bowl
Calories:	121	Fat:	4 grams
Carbohydrates:	6 grams	Protein:	12 grams
Fiber	4 grams		

Hamburger Veggie Soup

When money was getting low, my mom would always make hamburger soup. Hamburger was cheap and we always grew lots of vegetables in the garden. Mom's soup had noodles, but I just substituted long strands of cabbage for those noodles in this recipe.

Ingredients:

- 1 tablespoon olive oil

- 1-pound hamburger

- ½ large onion, peeled and diced

- ½ large green or red pepper, diced

- 2 stalks celery, diced

- 1 14-ounce can stewed or diced tomatoes

- 32 ounces chicken stock

- 1 teaspoon salt

- ½ teaspoon garlic powder

- 1 teaspoon apple cider vinegar

- 1 pinch of stevia powder

- ½ small cabbage, shredded

- Water as needed

Directions:

1. Heat a heavy skillet and add the olive oil. Add the hamburger and cook all the way through, breaking it up.

2. Drain the hamburger and place on a paper towel to get rid of any excess grease. Set aside.

3. Put a stock pot on the stove and add the onion, green pepper and celery and sauté about three minutes.

4. Add the tomatoes and chicken stock and simmer until the vegetables become tender.

5. Add the drained hamburger.

6. Add salt and pepper to taste as well as the garlic powder, vinegar, stevia, and cabbage.

7. Cook for 20 minutes or until the cabbage is tender.

8. If the soup boils down during those 20 minutes, add a little water or chicken stock.

9. Serve hot.

Good-for-You Cream of Broccoli Soup

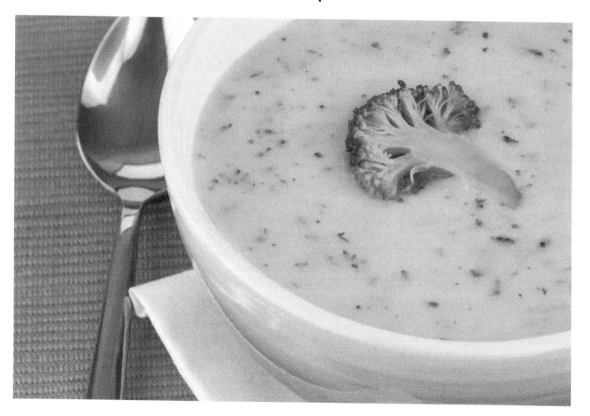

Nutritional Information Per Serving			
Yield:	4 servings	Serving Size:	1 bowl
Calories:	106	Fat:	6 grams
Carbohydrates:	24 grams	Protein:	10 grams
Fiber	8 grams		

Cream of Broccoli Soup

Regular cream of broccoli soup has loads of milk, but I have found a way to cut down on the dairy in this soup. I add cauliflower, which is a natural thickener. You blend everything together, making a creamy soup that is quite filling.

Ingredients:

- 1 tablespoon olive oil

- 1 rib celery, chopped small

- 1 small onion, peeled and diced

- 1 teaspoon salt

- ¼ teaspoon onion powder

- ¼ teaspoon garlic powder

- ½ teaspoon celery seed

- ¼ teaspoon white pepper

- 8 cups broccoli florets, divided

- 4 cups cauliflower florets

- 3 cups chicken broth

- 1 cup 2% milk

Directions:

86

1. Set a heavy stock pot on the stove over medium heat and add the olive oil.

2. Put in the celery, onion, and salt and sauté for three minutes or until softened and fragrant.

3. Add the onion powder, garlic powder, celery seed, white pepper, seven cups of broccoli, cauliflower, and chicken broth to the pot. Cover loosely and bring to a boil. Turn the heat down to a simmer for about 10 minutes or until the cauliflower is fork tender.

4. Place half of the hot soup in a blender and process it until smooth and creamy. Pour this liquid into a temporary container and proceed with the other half. You can also use an immersion blender, if you wish. Pour all the soup back into the stock pot and add the rest of the broccoli and milk.

5. Bring the pot up to a boil over medium heat. This will cook the rest of the broccoli and make the soup a little chunky. Once it starts to boil, turn off the heat and serve immediately.

Hearty Beef Stew

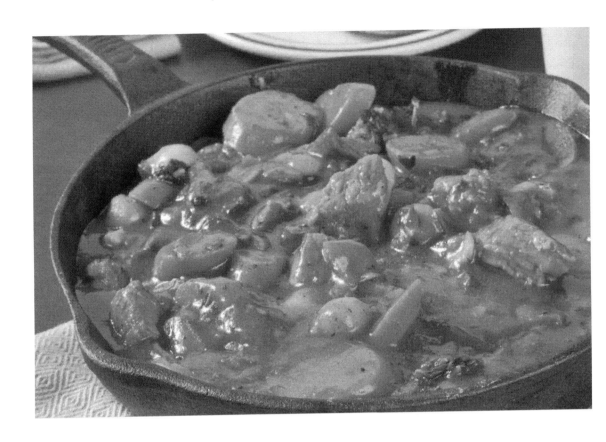

Nutritional Information Per Serving			
Yield:	4 servings	Serving Size:	1 bowl
Calories:	432	Fat:	36 grams
Carbohydrates:	6 grams	Protein:	19 grams
Fiber	2 grams		

Hearty Beef Stew

Beef stew is a staple at our house in the winter. This stew is a little different because it calls for radishes and the thickener is xanthan gum. I also used coconut oil instead of vegetable oil, for a slightly richer flavor.

Ingredients:

- 1 pound beef round steak

- ¼ teaspoon salt

- ¼ teaspoon pepper

- 1 tablespoon coconut oil

- 1 tablespoon butter

- 3 cloves garlic, minced

- ½ cup celery, chopped

- ½ cup carrot, peeled and chopped

- ½ cup onion, peeled and chopped

- 2 cups beef broth

- ½ teaspoon xanthan gum

- ½ cup radishes, chopped

Directions:

1. Cut the beef round steak into small, bite-sized pieces and toss with salt and pepper. Set aside.

2. Heat a large saucepan and add the coconut oil. Add the beef chunks and brown on all sides. Remove from the pot and set aside.

3. Melt the butter in the pan and add the garlic, celery, carrots, and onion. Sauté for a couple minutes, stirring constantly.

4. Add the broth and stir.

5. Add the xanthan gum and stir well. Bring to a boil, add meat, and reduce the heat to simmer for 30 minutes, stirring frequently. The xanthan gum will thicken the stew. If it becomes too thick, simply add a little water.

6. Add the radishes and cook another 30 minutes, stirring frequently. Add water as needed to maintain the ideal consistency.

7. Serve hot.

Noodle-less Chicken Soup

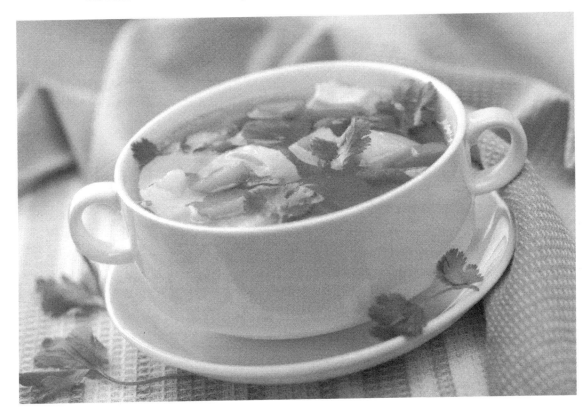

Nutritional Information Per Serving			
Yield:	4 servings	Serving Size:	large bowl
Calories:	197	Fat:	4 grams
Carbohydrates:	6 grams	Protein:	34 grams
Fiber	2 grams		

Noodle-less Chicken Soup

Okay, so you can't have chicken noodle soup, mainly because noodles are high in carbohydrates, but you can still have the soup part. If you fill up your soup with lots of vegetables, you might not even miss the noodles. This soup is hearty and satisfying.

Ingredients:

- 1 5- to 6-pound whole chicken

- 3 quarts water

- ½ large red onion, chopped

- 4 stalks of celery, chopped

- 4 cloves garlic, peeled and crushed

- 2 large carrots, peeled and chopped

- 2 sprigs fresh rosemary

- 3 sprigs fresh thyme

- ½ teaspoon salt

- ¼ teaspoon pepper

Directions:

1. Clean and cut up the chicken. Separate the breasts, legs, thighs, and wings and remove the skin from just the breasts.

2. Place water into a stock pot and place the chicken pieces in the water. Turn the heat on to medium high and bring the water to a boil.

3. Reduce the heat and simmer for 15 minutes.

4. Add the onion, celery, and garlic and simmer for 30 minutes.

5. Add the carrots, rosemary, thyme, salt, and pepper. Simmer for 30 more minutes.

6. The meat should be falling off the bones by now and the fat should be rising to the top of the pot. Skim as much of the fat off the top as possible. If you don't, you will have greasy soup. Once the fat is gone, extract the chicken with a slotted spoon.

7. Keep the soup simmering and wait until the chicken has cooled a little before you debone it. Chop the meat slightly and return it to the pot, simmering for 20 more minutes.

8. Serve hot.

Pork Chili Verdi (Green Chili Pork Stew)

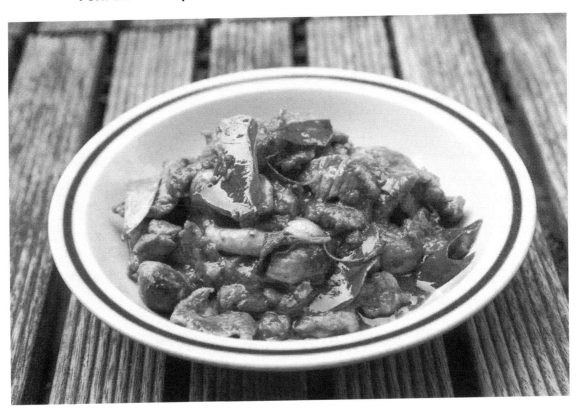

Nutritional Information Per Serving			
Yield:	8 servings	Serving Size:	1 bowl
Calories:	182	Fat:	10 grams
Carbohydrates:	4 grams	Protein:	20 grams
Fiber	1 gram		

Pork Chili Verdi

This recipe comes from my sister-in-law in New Mexico where she learned it from the locals. If you want to add a little Latin flair to your dinner, this is the dish for you.

Ingredients:

- 2 tablespoons olive oil

- 2 pounds pork loin, cut into bite-sized cubes

- 2 teaspoons garlic powder

- 2 teaspoons ground cumin

- 1 teaspoon chili powder

- 1 27-ounce can whole green chilies, liquid included

- 2 cloves garlic, peeled

- ½ cup onion, peeled and chopped

- 2 cups water

- 1 fried or poached egg for each serving (optional)

Directions:

1. In a large skillet, heat the oil and add the cubed pork loin. Add the garlic powder, cumin, and chili powder and brown on all sides. Turn the heat down and keep stirring so the pork does not burn.

2. While browning the pork, place the can of chilies and liquid in a blender or food processer along with the garlic cloves and onion. Process to make a chunky paste-like substance.

3. Pour the sauce over the pork and add the water. Stir well and turn the heat down to medium low. Cover the skillet leaving the lid ajar and simmer for 1½ hours or until the pork is tender. You may need to add a little water, so check every 15 to 20 minutes. Do not use broth or anything with salt; it will be salty enough.

4. Ladle stew into bowls and top with a hot fried or poached egg.

Pumpkin-Pork Stew à la Crock-Pot

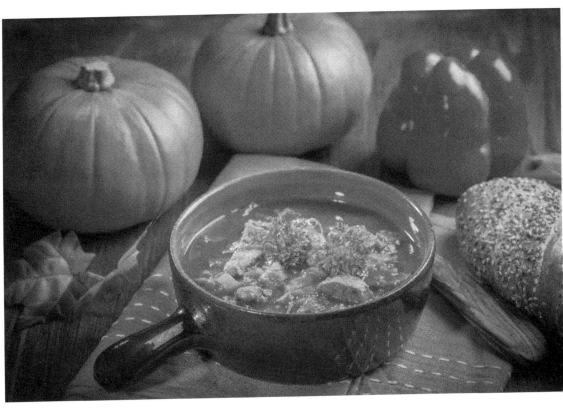

Nutritional Information Per Serving			
Yield:	6 servings	Serving Size:	1 bowl
Calories:	451	Fat:	33 grams
Carbohydrates:	4 grams	Protein:	28 grams
Fiber	0 grams		

Pumpkin Pork Stew

I simply *had* to include this recipe; it is unusual but oh, so delicious! I love pumpkin and used to only eat it in pie. Pumpkin is low-carb and perfect for the ketogenic diet. This recipe includes typical pumpkin pie spices and it is sweetened with a sugar substitute. To add to the interesting ingredients, it also contains habanero peppers and peanut butter. This may sound strange, but everything combines to make a delicious meal.

Ingredients:

- 2 pounds country style pork ribs without the bones

- ½ teaspoon salt

- ¼ teaspoon pepper

- 2 tablespoons olive oil, divided

- 1 clove garlic, peeled and minced

- 1 teaspoon fresh ginger, peeled and minced

- ½ teaspoon habanero pepper, minced

- 1 tablespoon smooth peanut butter

- ½ cup dry white wine

- 2 cups chicken stock

- 2 cups water

- ¼ cup stevia

95

- ¼ teaspoon ground allspice

- ¼ teaspoon ground cardamom

- 1 cup pumpkin puree

Directions:

1. Season the pork with salt and pepper. Heat a heavy frying pan and add one tablespoon of the olive oil. Sear the pork on all sides, but do not cook through. Place the pork in the bottom of a Crock-Pot that has been coated with non-stick spray.

2. Add the garlic, ginger, and habanero pepper to the frying pan, along with the rest of the olive oil and the peanut butter. Whisk together and cook for two to three minutes, until the onions soften.

3. Add the wine and let it bubble for about a minute.

4. Add the water, chicken stock, cardamom, allspice, sugar substitute, and pumpkin puree. Whisk it smooth and heat until it bubbles. Immediately pour over the pork in the crock pot.

5. Cook on high two hours or on low for four hours. The pork should fall apart, so shredding it will take almost no effort; just use a couple forks.

6. Ladle into bowls and serve while hot.

Rich, Heart-Warming Tomato Soup

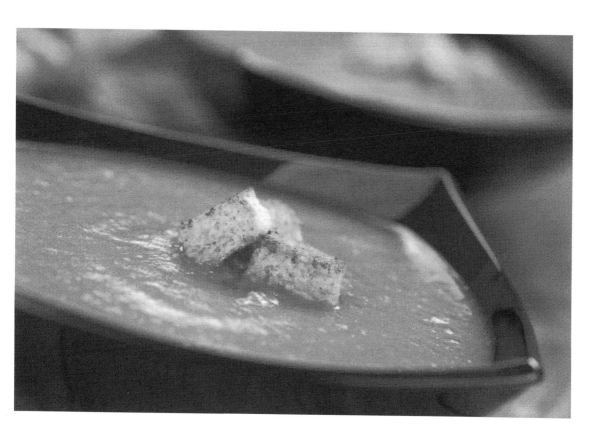

Nutritional Information Per Serving			
Yield:	4 servings	Serving Size:	1 bowl
Calories:	304	Fat:	28 grams
Carbohydrates:	57 grams	Protein:	13 grams
Fiber	1 grams		

Tomato Soup

Tomato soup is a comfort food from my childhood. My parents used to buy the red and white soup cans from the grocery store and when we came in from playing in the snow, this soup would be ready for us, steaming hot.

This version tastes a little more refined than the canned soup and it will please the adult palate quite nicely. The recipe includes

97

croutons made from cheddar cheese that give it an extra touch of elegance.

Ingredients:

- 1 cup shredded cheddar cheese

- ¼ teaspoon garlic powder

- 2 teaspoons olive oil

- 1 clove garlic, peeled and chopped fine

- 1 tablespoon finely chopped onion

- 1 28-ounce can crushed tomatoes

- 1 cup chicken broth

- ½ cup heavy whipping cream

- Salt and pepper to taste

- 2 tablespoons fresh basil, chopped

Directions:

1. Prepare a baking sheet by covering it with parchment paper and lightly coating with non-stick spray.

2. Preheat oven to 350 degrees Fahrenheit.

3. Take your shredded cheddar cheese and place it in small crouton-size mounds, spacing them about 1½ inches apart. Sprinkle each mound with the garlic powder.

4. Bake for five minutes, watching carefully so that the cheese mounds turn lightly brown at the edges but do not burn. Remove from the oven and set aside to cool.

5. Place a large pot over medium heat and pour in the olive oil.

6. Add the garlic and onions and sauté for about two to three minutes.

7. Add the tomatoes and simmer for 10 minutes.

8. Add the chicken broth and simmer for five minutes.

9. Turn the heat off and add the cream, whisking it in well. Add the salt and pepper to taste.

10. Pour into bowls, garnish with basil, and top with cheese croutons.

Chapter 5: Beef Recipes That Will Make Your Mouth Water

Beef Stroganoff With Zucchini Noodles

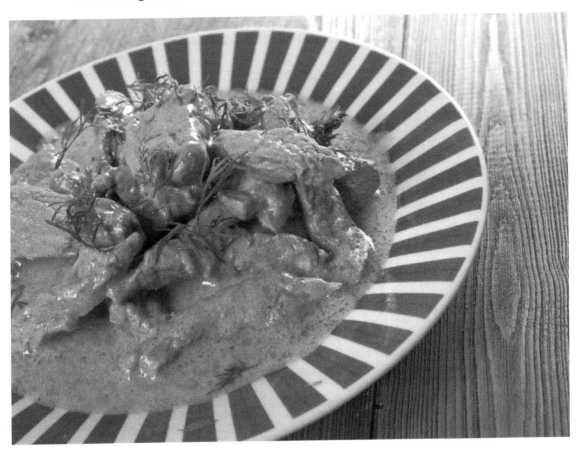

Nutritional Information Per Serving			
Yield:	4 servings	Serving Size:	~2 cups
Calories:	479	Fat:	14 grams
Carbohydrates:	22 grams	Protein:	66 grams
Fiber	7 grams		

Beef Stroganoff with Zucchini Noodles

Beef stroganoff is one of those meals you can dress up or down. It is naturally elegant but easy to make. This recipe uses zucchini strips in place of high-carb noodles. It calls for arrowroot flour to thicken the mix.

Ingredients:

- 1 tablespoon olive oil

- 2 pounds beef round steak, cut in half-inch strips

- 1 clove garlic, peeled and finely chopped

- 1 small onion, peeled and finely chopped

- ½ teaspoon sea salt

- ¼ teaspoon pepper

- 6 cups water, divided

- 2 tablespoons Dijon mustard

- 1 tablespoon fresh rosemary

- 2 cups mushrooms, quartered

- ½ cup frozen pearl onions

- ½ cup fat-free Greek yogurt

- 2 tablespoons arrowroot flour

- 1 tablespoon fresh parsley, finely chopped

- 8 small zucchinis, skin removed, cut in ribbons

Directions:

1. Heat a large pan or Dutch oven and add the olive oil. Sear the strips of meat on all sides.

2. Add the garlic, onion, salt, and pepper and lower burner to medium heat. Stir until the onions soften.

3. Add two cups of water, Dijon mustard, and rosemary, stirring until it combines well. Cover the pot loosely and lower to a simmer. Watch until almost all of the liquid evaporates, then add the other two cups of water. Let about half of this water also evaporate.

4. Add mushrooms and pearl onions, bringing the mixture to a boil.

5. Separately, mix together the yogurt, arrowroot flour, and ½ cup of liquid, drawn from the pot. Whisk to incorporate and add it back into the pan. Turn off the heat and stir well. The mixture should thicken quickly.

6. Add the parsley, cover, and set aside.

7. Serve over cooked and drained zucchini ribbons.

Cheese-Stuffed Bacon Burgers

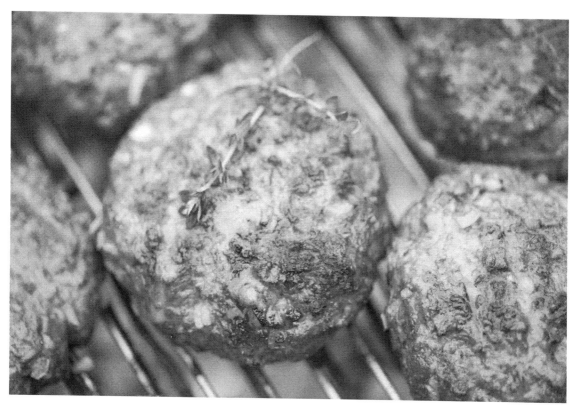

The burgers before the bacon

Nutritional Information Per Serving			
Yield:	4 servings	Serving Size:	1 burger
Calories:	615	Fat:	52 grams
Carbohydrates:	1.5 grams	Protein:	33 grams
Fiber	0 grams		

Cheese-Stuffed Bacon Burgers

At first glance, this is a normal cheeseburger with bacon on top. Yet, bite into it and you discover an entirely different cheesy flavor inside. You can grill this outdoors or cook it on the stove; either way, you get four juicy flavor bombs to enjoy.

Ingredients:

- 4 slices bacon

- 2 teaspoons of salt

- 1 teaspoon pepper

- 2 teaspoons Cajun seasoning

- 1-pound ground beef

- 4 ounces cheddar cheese (not shredded)

- 2 ounces Mozzarella cheese, divided

- 2 tablespoons butter

Directions:

1. Cook the bacon, cool it on paper towels, and set aside.

2. In a large bowl, combine the salt, pepper, Cajun seasoning, and ground beef. Mix well and set aside.

3. Cut the cheddar cheese into four slices and set aside.

4. Cube one ounce of the Mozzarella cheese.

5. Shape the ground beef into four patties and place some of the Mozzarella in the very center of each patty, folding the beef over it.

6. Heat the butter in a skillet and once it is bubbling, add the burgers. Turn the heat to medium low, place a cover over the skillet, and let it cook for two to three minutes.

7. Remove the lid, flip the burgers, and cook them covered, for another two minutes.

8. Flip the burgers again and place a slice of cheddar cheese atop each patty, then cover and cook for another one to two minutes until melted.

9. Break up the bacon slices and sprinkle them on top of the burgers, then serve.

Crock-Pot Beef Pot Roast

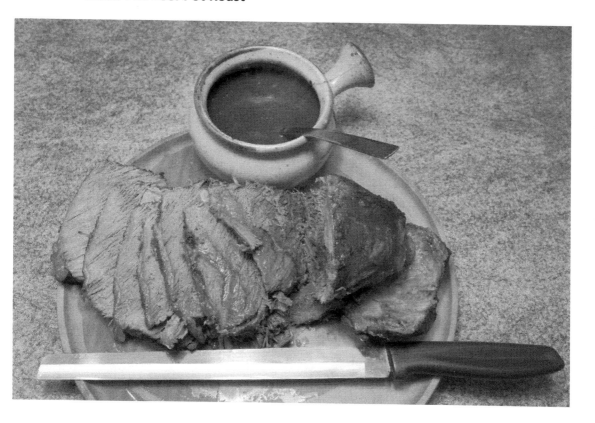

Nutritional Information Per Serving			
Yield:	4 patties	Serving Size:	1 patty
Calories:	499	Fat:	23 grams
Carbohydrates:	0 grams	Protein:	63 grams
Fiber	0 grams		

Beef Pot Roast

Everyone should have a "go to" pot roast recipe; this is mine. It is cooked in a Crock-Pot; I put it on in the morning and when I come home at the end of the day, it is ready to go. Regular pot roast recipes contain potatoes and vegetables, but this one is *just* the pot roast. You can probably throw in some carrots and cauliflower if you want, but you will have to adjust the nutritional numbers.

Ingredients:

Seasoning rub:

- 1½ teaspoons salt

- 1 teaspoon garlic powder

- ¼ teaspoon thyme

- ¼ teaspoon oregano

- ¼ teaspoon rosemary

- ¼ teaspoon parsley

- ¼ teaspoon basil

Other **Ingredients:**

- 2 tablespoons olive oil

- 1 2½-pound boneless chuck roast

- 2 strips bacon

- 1 cup beef broth

- ¼ cup apple cider vinegar

- 2 tablespoons tomato paste

- ¼ teaspoon salt

- 1 small onion, peeled and chopped

- 4 stalks celery, chopped

- 2 cloves garlic, peeled and minced

- 2 bay leaves

Directions:

1. In a small bowl, combine the rub ingredients and rub them all over the roast. Set aside.

2. Heat olive oil in a large Dutch oven. Place the roast in and brown evenly on all sides, including the ends.

3. Transfer the roast into a Crock-Pot treated with non-stick spray and set the bacon on top.

4. Pour the broth around the edges of the roast.

5. In a bowl, whisk the vinegar with the tomato paste and salt. Pour this mixture around the sides of the Crock-Pot.

6. Place the onion, celery, and garlic on top of the roast and lay the bay leaves over all.

7. Pour any liquid in the Dutch oven into the crock pot.

8. Cook on high for three to four hours or on low for eight hours.

9. Remove the bay leaves before serving.

Greek-Inspired Beef Zucchini Burgers

Nutritional Information Per Serving			
Yield:	6 servings	Serving Size:	2 burgers
Calories:	349	Fat:	20 grams
Carbohydrates:	3.5grams	Protein:	35 grams
Fiber	0.6 grams		

This recipe has a lovely feta cheese sauce that is to die for. It is very easy to make and gets rid of a craving for burgers, even though you eat it with a fork.

Ingredients:

- 1½ cups zucchini, grated

- 1½ pounds ground beef

- ½ teaspoon salt

- ¼ teaspoon pepper

- ½ teaspoon cinnamon

- 2 teaspoons cumin

- 5 ounces feta cheese, divided

- ½ cup sour cream

- 2 tablespoons lemon juice, fresh squeezed

- Lettuce leaves

Directions:

1. In a bowl, mix the zucchini with the beef. Add salt, pepper, cinnamon, and cumin. Form the mixture into 12 small burgers and set aside.

2. Grill the burgers until both sides are brown and they are almost done. Transfer to a skillet and cook another five to eight minutes or until done (5 minutes for medium well and eight for well-done).

3. In a bowl whisk together four ounces of feta cheese and the sour cream. Stir in the lemon juice and set aside.

4. Place a lettuce leaf on a plate and top with two burgers. Crumble the rest of the feta cheese on top and drizzle three tablespoons of the sauce over each burger.

Green Bean And Hamburger Skillet

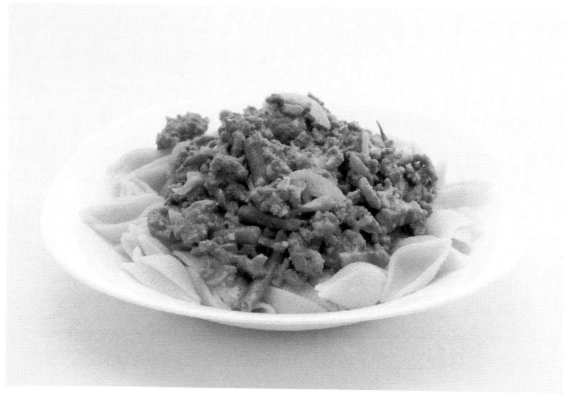

I cheated with pasta, but just this once!

Nutritional Information Per Serving

Yield:	4 servings	Serving Size:	½ cup
Calories:	244	Fat:	11 grams
Carbohydrates:	7 grams	Protein:	31 grams
Fiber	2 grams		

Green Bean Hamburger Skillet (no pasta)

This recipe will satisfy for a quick dinner. It is all made in one skillet in record time.

Ingredients:

- 1 tablespoon olive oil

- 2 cloves garlic, peeled and minced

- 1 pound hamburger

- ½ cup sliced water chestnuts, drained

- 1 8-ounce package frozen cut green beans, thawed and drained

- 2 tablespoons coconut amino sauce

Directions:

1. Heat a skillet over medium high heat and add the olive oil.

2. Add the garlic and sauté for one to two minutes.

3. Add the hamburger and brown well. Drain any fat that accumulates.

4. Add the water chestnuts and green beans and stir to incorporate.

5. Bring to a bubble and sprinkle the amino sauce over the mixture. Continue to cook until all is heated through.

6. Serve hot.

Keto Roasted Brisket

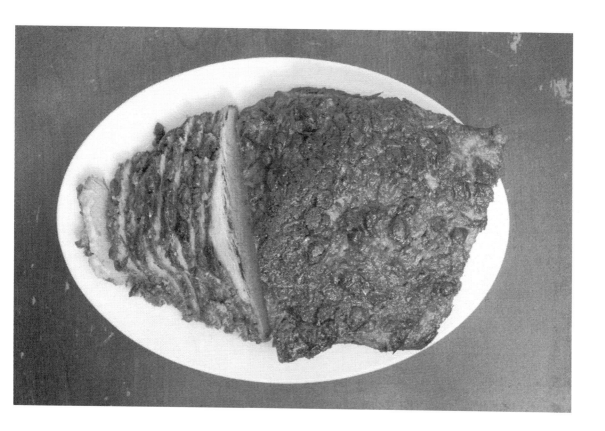

Nutritional Information Per Serving			
Yield:	varies	Serving Size:	4 ounces
Calories:	340	Fat:	22 grams
Carbohydrates:	0 grams	Protein:	32 grams
Fiber	0 grams		

Brisket

Brisket can come out dry and tough if it is very lean. Here is one situation where you want your brisket to have plenty of fat. It is also better to find grass-fed beef from a butcher or farm because it will not be as tough. Be careful NOT to get corned beef brisket.

This recipe cooks the brisket very slowly, so the flavor comes out and the brisket stays tender. Watch it during the last 45 minutes of cooking to ensure it is not drying out. If necessary, add water to keep the brisket moist.

Ingredients:

- ¼ teaspoon garlic powder

- ¼ teaspoon onion powder

- ¼ teaspoon salt

- ½ teaspoon pepper

- ¼ teaspoon dill seed

- ¼ teaspoon celery seed

- 1 4- to 5-pound beef brisket

Directions:

1. Preheat the oven to 350 degrees Fahrenheit.

2. In a bowl, mix the garlic powder, onion powder, salt pepper, dill seed, and celery seed. Sprinkle it all over the brisket.

3. Place the brisket in a baking dish and cover securely with foil.

4. Bake for one hour.

5. Reduce oven to 300 degrees Fahrenheit and remove the brisket from the oven.

6. Pour a half inch of hot water into the pan around the roast. Cover once more with foil and set it back in the oven for two hours, then check it. If the water is less than a quarter inch deep, add more water to replace what evaporated. Cook for two to three more hours.

7. The brisket is done when it reaches 140 degrees internally on a meat thermometer. Remove from the pan and let it set on a cutting board for 10 minutes before slicing.

8. Thicken the juices with your desired thickening agent and serve as gravy.

Ketogenic Steak

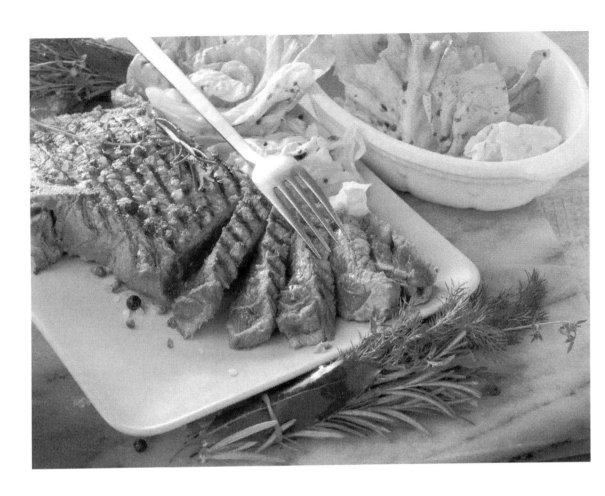

Nutritional Information Per Serving			
Yield:	4 servings	Serving Size:	½ steak
Calories:	700	Fat:	30 grams
Carbohydrates:	0 grams	Protein:	41 grams
Fiber	0 grams		

Steak

Sometimes you just want a steak, after all it's naturally ketogenic! Whenever you hanker for a steak, this recipe will deliver what you desire. The recipe is simple and quick. It uses ghee instead of oil. Ghee is a clarified butter that is most often used in the cuisines of India, Africa, and the Middle East. You can find it at a Middle Eastern grocery or a health food store.

You will cook this in a shallow baking dish with a rack inside it. The steaks I prefer to use are either large strip or ribeye steaks. I have tried this with filet mignon, but they take much longer to cook. The steaks should be about 1½-inches thick and a bit over 1½ pounds in weight. They are cut into four servings. The best part: steak has no carbs whatsoever.

Ingredients:

- 2 boneless steaks (see above for size)

- Sea salt and cracked pepper to taste

- 2 tablespoons ghee

Directions:

1. Preheat the oven to 275 degrees Fahrenheit.

2. Pat the steaks dry with a paper towel and cut in half to make four evenly sized steaks.

3. Smear all sides with ghee and season with salt and pepper.

4. Place on a wire rack set inside a rimmed baking dish that has been lined with foil.

5. Put in the oven and cook for 20 to 25 minutes or until the internal temperature reaches 90 to 95 degrees, Fahrenheit, for rare. Leave in a little longer for medium or boost the temperature by 10 degrees Fahrenheit to cook more thoroughly in the same amount of time.

6. Heat a large skillet and add the ghee over high heat. Introduce the steak pieces and cook for one to two minutes on each side. You'll want to keep ghee between the pan and the steak in order to slightly caramelize the meat.

7. Place on a clean wire rack, cover loosely with foil and let rest for 10 minutes before serving.

Sesame Beef And Daikon Stir Fry

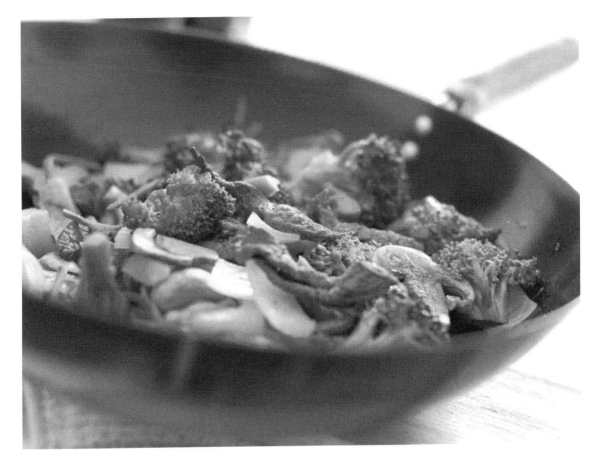

Nutritional Information Per Serving			
Yield:	4 servings	Serving Size:	1½ cups
Calories:	349	Fat:	31 grams
Carbohydrates:	5 grams	Protein:	25 grams
Fiber	0.1 gram		

Sesame Beef Daikon Stir-Fry

Daikon is a Japanese winter radish; it is usually white in color and has a mild radish flavor. I love daikon, so whenever I see a recipe that uses it, I try it out. This one did not disappoint.

In this recipe, the daikon radish is used in place of the usual noodles. Since a ketogenic diet rules out the use of noodles made from most types of flour, you'll find all sorts of things pressed into service as replacements in these recipes.

Stir frying is a rapid cooking method, using high heat. You can prepare a stir-fried meal in just a few seconds. Of course, this calls for a little prep time, chopping up the contents beforehand. I often chop up everything the night before and refrigerate the various ingredients in individual bags. All I need to do the next day is drop the contents into a hot wok or saucepan and stir while they cook. When everything's pre-prepped, I can get this meal on the table in mere minutes.

This recipe calls for a couple atypical **Ingredients:** coconut flour and guar gum. Both are readily available in health food stores and are starting to show up in grocery stores as well. The recipe also includes a bunch of spicy ingredients, so prepare your taste buds; it will really wake them up.

Ingredients:

- 1 medium daikon radish (¼ pound)

- Water

- 1 tablespoon coconut flour

- ½ teaspoon guar gum

- 1 pound ribeye steak, cut in thin strips

- 1 tablespoon coconut oil

- 1 clove garlic, peeled and minced

117

- 1 teaspoon ginger, peeled and minced

- ½ Jalapeno pepper, seeded and sliced in thin rings

- ½ red pepper, seeded and sliced in thin rings

- 2 green onions, chopped

- ¼ teaspoon red pepper flakes

- 3 tablespoons coconut amino sauce

- 1 teaspoon oyster sauce

- 1 teaspoon sesame oil

- 1 teaspoon rice vinegar

- 6 drops liquid stevia

- 1-inch coconut oil

- 1 tablespoon toasted sesame seeds

Directions:

1. Either use a spiral slicer to slice the daikon into noodle-like strings, or use a vegetable peeler to cut thin strips. Soak in a bowl of cold water for 20 minutes.

2. In a bowl, mix the coconut flour and guar gum. Coat the ribeye strips and let them set for 10 minutes.

3. In a wok, heat the coconut oil. Add the garlic, ginger, jalapeño, bell pepper, onion, and red pepper flakes. Stir fry for two to three minutes.

4. In a bowl, whisk together the coconut amino sauce, oyster sauce, sesame oil, rice vinegar, and liquid sweetener. Add this to the wok and stir fry for two more minutes.

5. While cooking in the wok, heat the cooking oil in a large pot until it reaches 325 degrees Fahrenheit.

6. Place the beef in the oil, a little at a time, and fry for three minutes on each side or until it shows a brown crust. Drain on paper towels.

7. Place the meat in the wok and stir fry for two more minutes.

8. Drain the daikon slices, and place them on serving plates. Top with the beef mixture and sprinkle with sesame seeds before serving.

Slow-Cooked Beef And Broccoli Stir Fry

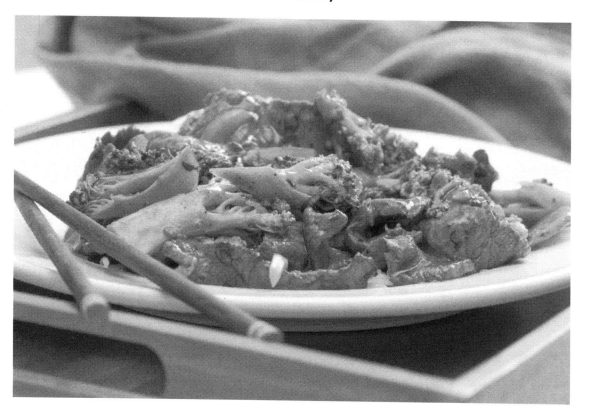

Nutritional Information Per Serving

Yield:	4 servings	Serving Size:	~1 cup
Calories:	430	Fat:	19 grams
Carbohydrates:	4 grams	Protein:	54 grams
Fiber	1 gram		

Beef-Broccoli Stir Fry

This slow cooker recipe is very easy to make. You can be sitting down to eat within 30 minutes of arriving home. This recipe includes coconut aminos, a wonderful low-carb alternative for soy sauce. It can be found at any health food store.

Ingredients:

- 2 pounds flank steak

- 1 cup beef broth

- ⅔ cup coconut aminos

- 3 tablespoons stevia

- 3 cloves garlic, peeled and minced

- 1 teaspoon ginger, peeled and grated

- ¼ teaspoon red pepper flakes

- ½ teaspoon salt

- 1 head broccoli, cut into florets

- 1 red bell pepper, seeded and cut in 1-inch chunks

- 1 teaspoon sesame seeds

Directions:

1. Prepare the Crock-Pot by coating with a nonstick spray and turning it on low.

2. Cut the flank steak into two-inch chunks or strips.

3. Place the steak in the Crock-Pot and top with the beef broth, coconut aminos, sweetener, garlic, red pepper flakes, and salt.

4. Cover and cook on low for five to six hours.

5. Stir the ingredients in the Crock-Pot, then add the broccoli and red pepper chunks on top and cover again. Cook for 30 minutes on high heat.

6. Sprinkle with sesame seeds and serve. You can serve by itself or atop riced cauliflower (not included in the nutritional totals).

Note: If the mixture is too watery, you can create a slurry using one tablespoon of arrowroot flour to two tablespoons of cold water. Add this after the broccoli and peppers have cooked. It should thicken quickly.

Steak Pinwheels

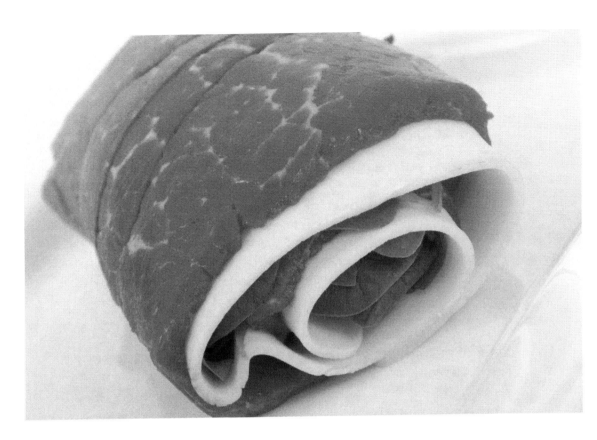

I used mozzarella slices here and thin-sliced mea; the roll before tying and baking.

Nutritional Information Per Serving			
Yield:	6 servings	Serving Size:	1 pinwheel
Calories:	519	Fat:	29 grams
Carbohydrates:	1 grams	Protein:	57 grams
Fiber	1 gram		

Steak Pinwheels

This is another elegant recipe you can easily serve on special occasions or enjoy every day. The pinwheels are quite beautiful, with cheese and spinach rolled up and sliced to expose the colorful layers.

Ingredients:

- 1 2½-pound flank steak

- 2 to 3 teaspoons Italian seasoning

- 16 ounces shredded Mozzarella cheese

- 8 ounces fresh spinach leaves

Directions:

1. Preheat the oven to 350 degrees Fahrenheit.

2. Butterfly the flank steak.

3. Season both sides of the steak with the Italian seasoning.

4. Add a thin layer of fresh spinach leaves over a non-stick sprayed glass casserole dish and set aside.

5. Spread the shredded Mozzarella on the meat, leaving one inch plain on one side for wrapping.

6. Lay down a layer of spinach leaves over the cheese.

7. Roll up the flank steak, keeping it tight and rolling with the grain of the meat.

8. Cut six pieces of cooking twine and tie the roll evenly so that the twine will be in the middle of a slice. Use a sharp knife to cut into six pieces with the twine in the middle of the slice.

9. Lay the slices atop the spinach.

10. Bake for 25 minutes or until the meat is the desired doneness.

11. Place under the broiler for three minutes to cause the Mozzarella cheese to bubble, then serve.

Beef supplies you with a great deal of protein, probably more than any other meat, but you can't live on beef alone. The following chapter introduces a variety of poultry dishes that utilize chicken, turkey, and even duck.

Chapter 6: World Class Poultry Recipes

I love to cook with chicken because it is so versatile. I have included a few casseroles and other chicken dishes that are traditional and delicious. In this chapter, you'll find a turkey pot pie with a special ketogenic crust. I have even included a delicious turkey tetrazzini. I am not a fan of duck, but a friend gave me permission to use her favorite recipe; I hope you like it

Breaded Parmesan Bacon Chicken

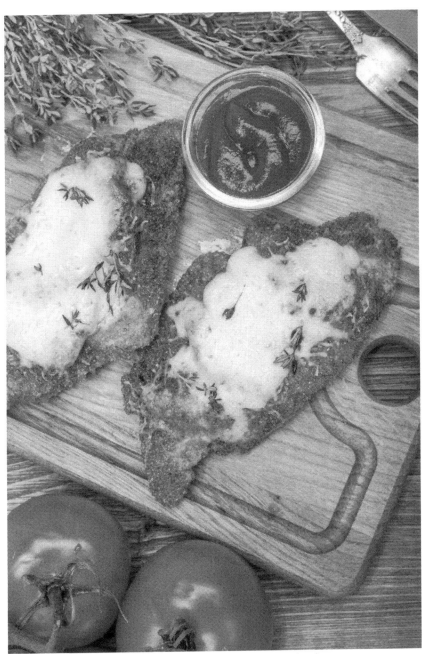

I melted the cheese before adding the bacon.

Nutritional Information Per Serving

Yield:	4 servings	Serving Size:	1 piece
Calories:	413	Fat:	23 grams
Carbohydrates:	1 grams	Protein:	49 grams
Fiber	0 grams		

Breaded Parmesan Bacon Chicken

Yes, this is breaded Parmesan chicken, but we use cheese for the breading, instead of carb-laden bread.

Ingredients:

- 1 egg, beaten

- 1 tablespoon water

- ½ teaspoon salt

- 1 cup Parmesan cheese

- ¼ teaspoon garlic powder

- ¼ teaspoon black pepper

- 4 boneless chicken breasts

- ½ cup olive oil

- 1½ cups Asiago cheese, shredded

- 4 slices bacon, cooked and crumbled

Directions:

1. Preheat the oven to 350 degrees Fahrenheit.

2. In a bowl, mix the egg with the water until well combined and set aside.

3. In another bowl, combine the Parmesan cheese, salt, pepper, and garlic.

4. Dip each chicken breast in the egg and then in the cheese mixture.

5. In a skillet, add the oil and wait until it gets hot. If it isn't hot enough, the breading will stick to the pan and not the chicken. Fry each chicken breast until it is golden brown.

6. Line a baking pan with foil and fit a wire rack on top. Place the browned chicken on the rack and slide it in the oven.

7. Cook about 20 minutes, until the juices run clear. Remove from the oven and turn on the broiler.

8. Top each breast with Asiago cheese and a strip of bacon, then slide the pan under the broiler to melt the cheese.

9. Serve immediately.

Chicken Parmesan Casserole

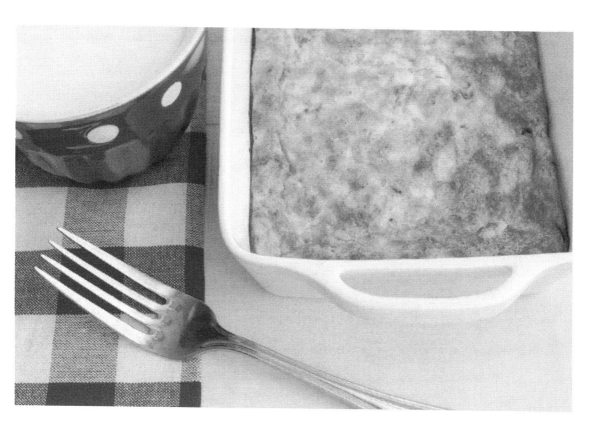

Nutritional Information Per Serving			
Yield:	8 servings	Serving Size:	1 piece
Calories:	302	Fat:	8 grams
Carbohydrates:	8 grams	Protein:	28 grams
Fiber	2 grams		

Chicken Parmesan Casserole

I used to buy a perfectly scrumptious chicken Parmesan sandwich at my favorite restaurant. It had a breaded chicken breast, smothered with Italian sauce, and covered in Mozzarella cheese on a bun. The sandwich was wrapped in foil and baked until it was a delicious gooey mess.

On the ketogenic diet, flour breading and buns are taboo, but I found a casserole that will give you much of the flavor of my favorite sandwich. This recipe is highly versatile; it works just as well with boneless pork chops or even eggplant. Spaghetti squash substitutes for recipe's usual pasta. If you prefer, you can even swap out the squash for zucchini ribbons.

Ingredients:

- 1½ pounds boneless chicken breasts

- 1 egg

- ¼ cup grated Parmesan cheese

- ½ cup almond flour

- ¼ teaspoon sea salt

- ⅛ teaspoon black pepper

- ½ teaspoon dried basil

- ½ teaspoon garlic powder

- 3 tablespoons olive oil

- 4 cups cooked spaghetti squash, drained

- 1 tablespoon olive oil

- ¼ teaspoon sea salt

- ⅛ teaspoon black pepper

- ½ tablespoon dried parsley

- 1½ cups low sugar marinara sauce

- 6 ounces Mozzarella cheese, fresh, not shredded

- Fresh basil for garnish

Directions:

1. Cut the chicken breasts into bite-sized pieces and set aside.

2. Beat the egg in a small bowl and set aside.

3. In another bowl, whisk together the Parmesan cheese, almond flour, salt, pepper, dried basil, and garlic powder.

4. Dip the chicken pieces in egg and then dredge in the breading mixture.

5. Heat a non-stick sauté pan over medium heat and pour in the oil; add the chicken pieces and cook until both sides are golden. Drain on a paper towel and set aside.

6. Place the cooked spaghetti squash in a bowl and add the olive oil, salt, pepper, and parsley. Toss until the squash cum pasta is well coated.

7. Prepare an 8 by 12-inch baking dish with nonstick spray and spread the squash over the bottom.

8. Place a layer of chicken pieces over the top.

9. Spoon the marinara sauce on top of it all, making sure to cover the entire surface.

10. Cut the Mozzarella cheese into slices and lay it on top of the sauce.

11. Bake in a preheated 375-degree Fahrenheit oven for about 30 minutes or until the cheese is melted and the casserole is heated through.

12. Garnish with chopped fresh basil, cut into eight pieces, and serve hot.

Juicy Lemon Pepper Chicken

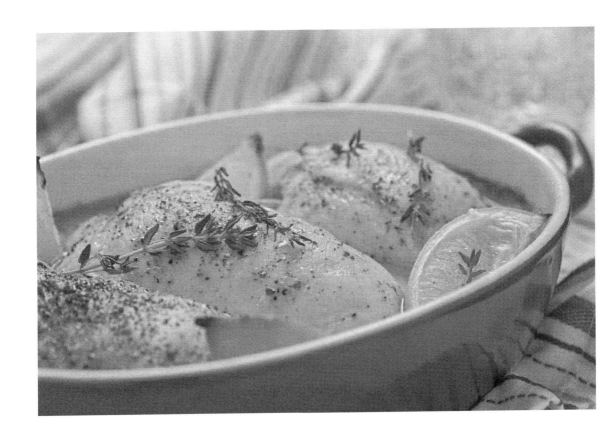

Nutritional Information Per Serving			
Yield:	6 servings	Serving Size:	1 piece
Calories:	336	Fat:	24 grams
Carbohydrates:	5 grams	Protein:	26 grams
Fiber	2 grams		

Baked Lemon Pepper Chicken

This recipe is made with three fresh lemons, making it luscious and lemony with a touch of pepper. The chicken is rich and juicy and it is one of the easiest recipes to make, with only four ingredients to deal with.

Ingredients:

- 1 whole 3-pound chicken, cut into pieces (breasts alone, if desired)

- 2 medium-sized lemons that have been juiced and zested (Keep the zest separate and reserve the lemon rinds.)

- ¼ teaspoon salt

- 2 tablespoons fresh ground black pepper

Directions:

1. Preheat the oven to 375 degrees Fahrenheit.

2. Line a 9 by 13-inch pan with foil and treat with nonstick spray.

3. Place the chicken pieces in the pan and pour the lemon juice over the top.

4. Sprinkle with salt, lemon zest, and pepper.

5. Place the cut-up lemon rind around and under the chicken pieces.

6. Bake, uncovered for 30 to 45 minutes, basting twice with the liquid that forms in the pan. The chicken juices should run clear when done.

7. Discard the lemon rind before serving.

Ketogenic Chicken Alfredo Casserole

Nutritional Information Per Serving			
Yield:	20 servings	Serving Size:	~1 cup
Calories:	549	Fat:	40 grams
Carbohydrates:	7 grams	Protein:	44 grams
Fiber	2 grams		

Most chicken Alfredo casserole recipes are loaded with high-carb pasta. To minimize the carbs, I replaced the pasta with low-carb vegetables. I usually use a bottled Alfredo sauce, but this recipe has enough portions for a crowd, so I included directions for making your own Alfredo sauce.

There are about 20 servings in this recipe. You can cut the recipe in half if you like, but a better idea is to make the whole thing and then freeze half. It freezes well and you'll just defrost the casserole when you want more and put it in the oven to bake.

Ingredients:

- 3½ pounds boneless, skinless chicken breasts

- ¼ teaspoon sea salt

- ¼ teaspoon pepper

- ½ teaspoon Italian seasoning

- 9 tablespoons olive oil, divided

- 6 tablespoons butter

- 3 cloves garlic, peeled and minced

- 6 cups heavy cream

- ¼ cup dried parsley

- ¾ cup grated Parmesan cheese

- ½ cup shredded Mozzarella cheese

- 32 ounces fresh cauliflower, chopped

- 32 ounces fresh broccoli, chopped

- 16 ounces fresh Mozzarella cheese, sliced

Directions:

Alfredo sauce:

1. Melt six tablespoons of olive oil along with the butter in a medium-sized saucepan over low heat.

2. Add the garlic, cream, and parsley and bring it to a simmer, stirring constantly.

3. Add the grated Parmesan cheese and the shredded Mozzarella; stir until the sauce thickens. You might need an immersion blender to reach a creamy consistency.

Casserole:

4. Sprinkle the salt, pepper, and Italian seasoning over the chicken.

5. Cook the chicken breasts in three tablespoons of the olive oil until cooked through. Set aside and let cool so you won't burn your hands when you cut it into bite-sized pieces.

6. Parboil the cauliflower and broccoli pieces until tender crisp and drain while making the sauce.

7. Cover an 11 by 15-inch baking pan with nonstick spray. Arrange the drained broccoli and cauliflower in the bottom and top with the chopped chicken.

8. Pour the sauce over all and top everything with sliced Mozzarella cheese.

9. Bake in a preheated 350-degree Fahrenheit oven for 45 to 55 minutes or until bubbly and browned. Serve hot.

Low-Carb Turkey Tetrazzini

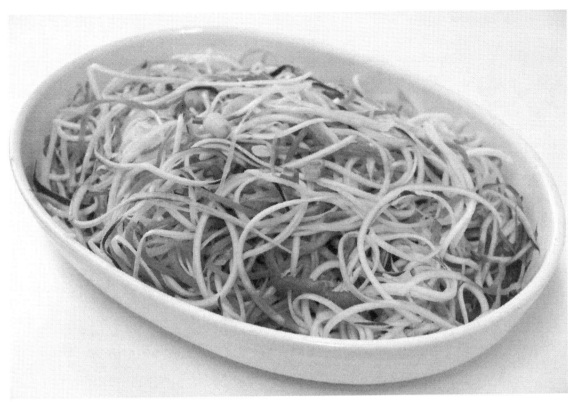

My zucchini-carrot noodle mix ready for the turkey mixture.

Nutritional Information Per Serving			
Yield:	8 servings	Serving Size:	1 piece
Calories:	270	Fat:	18 grams
Carbohydrates:	3 grams	Protein:	26 grams
Fiber	1 gram		

Low-Carb Turkey Tetrazzini

Turkey Tetrazzini is normally served over noodles, but in this recipe, I use zucchini noodles. There is a product on the market called Miracle Noodles, so-called because they are low carb; you can use them here if you can find them.

Ingredients:

- 4 cups zucchini noodles

136

- ½ cup cream cheese

- ½ cup chicken broth

- 1 egg, beaten

- 1 cup Parmesan cheese, grated

- 2 cups cheddar cheese, shredded and divided

- ¼ teaspoon garlic powder

- 1 teaspoon poultry seasoning

- ¼ teaspoon ground pepper

- 3 cups cabbage, shredded

- 3 cups cooked turkey that has been diced

Directions:

1. Preheat the oven to 400 degrees Fahrenheit and coat a 9 by 13-inch casserole dish with nonstick spray.

2. Peel the zucchini and cut into ribbons or noodles. Place in a colander and rinse with warm water. Set aside and drain well.

3. Mix the cream cheese, chicken broth, and beaten egg together in a large saucepan. Turn the heat to medium and once it melts together add the Parmesan cheese, 1½ cups of cheddar cheese, garlic powder, poultry seasoning, and pepper. Mix until it melts. Do not boil.

4. Add the cabbage and the turkey and remove from the burner.

5. Place zucchini noodles in the bottom of the baking dish, pour the turkey mixture on top, and cover the dish with foil.

6. Bake for 25 minutes, then remove the foil and sprinkle with the rest of the cheddar cheese. Return, uncovered, to the oven for 10 more minutes, then remove and let it set for 10 minutes.

7. Cut into eight pieces and serve hot.

NOTE: You can add other vegetables as well, but remember to adjust the nutritional values if you do.

Not-So-Old-Fashioned Turkey Pot Pie

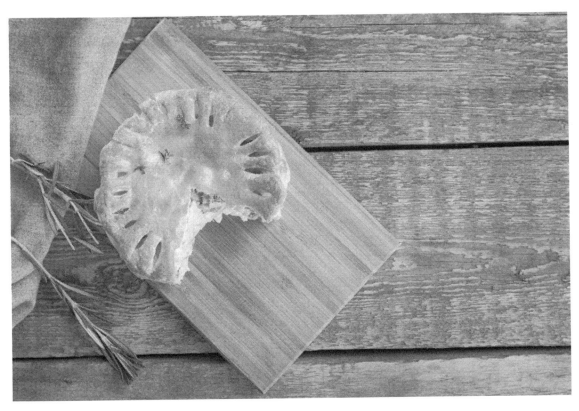

Nutritional Information Per Serving

Yield:	16 servings	Serving Size:	1 piece
Calories:	462	Fat:	40 grams
Carbohydrates:	9 grams	Protein:	21 grams
Fiber	2 grams		

Keto Turkey Pot Pie

A crust will add carbs to any recipe, but this crust is different. It is made from eggs, cream of tartar, and cream cheese. It has a different texture from regular pie crust, but it is still pretty good. This recipe will make two pies. You can freeze one, unbaked, for later if you want; just let it defrost in the refrigerator for a day, then pop it in the oven to bake for 30 minutes before dinner.

Ingredients:

- 3 eggs, separated

- ⅛ teaspoon cream of tartar

- 3 ounces cream cheese

- 6 tablespoons olive oil

- 6 tablespoons butter

- 3 cloves garlic, peeled and minced

- 6 cups heavy cream

- ¼ cup dried parsley

- ¾ cup grated Parmesan cheese

- ½ cup shredded Mozzarella cheese

- 2 cups cooked turkey

- 4 cups frozen mixed vegetables, thawed and drained

- ¼ cup Parmesan cheese

139

- 1 cup shredded Mozzarella cheese

Directions:

Alfredo Sauce:

1. Melt six tablespoons of olive oil along with the butter in a medium-sized saucepan over low heat.

2. Add the garlic, cream, and parsley and bring it to a simmer while stirring.

3. Add the grated Parmesan cheese and the shredded Mozzarella and stir until the sauce thickens. You might need an immersion blender to get a creamy consistency.

The Pot Pie:

4. Preheat the oven to 300 degrees Fahrenheit.

5. In a bowl, beat the egg whites with the cream of tartar until stiff peaks form, then set aside.

6. In another mixing bowl, beat the cream cheese with the egg yolks until smooth. Fold the egg whites into the cream cheese mixture carefully until just blended.

7. Pour the crust batter into two greased 9-inch pie pans. Put in oven for 30 minutes, remove, and let cool.

8. Preheat the oven to 350 degrees Fahrenheit.

9. Combine the Alfredo sauce, turkey, and vegetables in a bowl, then pour half into one crust and half into the other.

10. Combine the Parmesan and Mozzarella cheeses and sprinkle over the top of both pies.

11. Bake for 30 minutes or until the pie becomes bubbly and the cheese melts on top.

12. Let cool for five minutes, cut into wedges, and serve.

Pan-Seared Duck À L'Orange Over Wilted Spinach

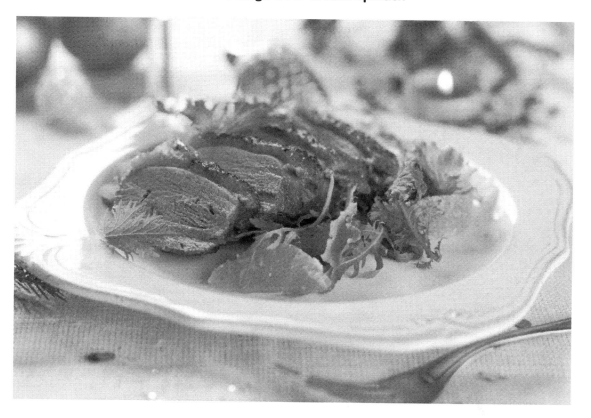

Nutritional Information Per Serving			
Yield:	1 serving	Serving Size:	1 duck breast
Calories:	798	Fat:	71 grams
Carbohydrates:	1.1 grams	Protein:	36 grams
Fiber	0.7 grams		

Duck à L'Orange over Wilted Spinach

I find duck a little intimidating to cook. I don't necessarily like rare meat and duck breast is best served a little on the rare side. Duck fat is also unusual. The skin is scored because it helps release the fat and makes the skin crispy and delicious.

In this recipe, a creamy orange sauce is made while the duck is rendering in another pan and then you put everything together. Duck cooks best in a steel pan rather than a non-stick pan; it makes the skin extra crispy. It is best to start with a cold pan as well, so that the fat renders from the breast correctly.

This recipe makes one serving only and it is best to cook each serving separately, a little underdone, then put all the servings in a preheated 300-degree oven for a few minutes to finish.

This is a high-calorie dish. If you are watching your calories, you can always reduce the size of the breast or only eat half of a serving.

Ingredients:

- I 6-ounce duck breast

- Salt and pepper to taste

- 2 tablespoons butter

- 1 tablespoon artificial sweetener

- ½ teaspoon dried sage

- ¼ teaspoon orange extract

- 1 tablespoon heavy cream

- 1 cup fresh spinach leaves

Directions:

1. Bring the breast to room temperature before beginning.

2. Pat the breast dry with a paper towel.

3. With a sharp knife, score the skin on the top side of the breast in a cross-hatch that goes less than an inch deep.

4. Season both sides of the breast with salt and pepper.

5. Place the duck breast, skin side down, in a cold stainless steel skillet and warm over medium heat. The fat will quickly start coming out of the breast. Tip the skillet periodically to remove the fat with a spoon into a heatproof container.

6. Cook the breast for about six minutes, then flip it over and cook another four minutes. The breast is done when it feels firm, yet springy when pushed on the top fleshy part with a finger.

7. Combine the heavy cream and the duck fat you have rendered from the breast and whisk well.

8. Pour the cream sauce over the duck and let it cook for a couple minutes over medium-low heat.

9. Wilt the spinach in the pan the cream sauce was in.

10. Place a bed of wilted spinach on a plate. Remove the duck from the heat and let it rest for five minutes before slicing. Arrange the slices on the spinach and pour sauce over the top.

Simply Smashing Stuffed Chicken Rolls

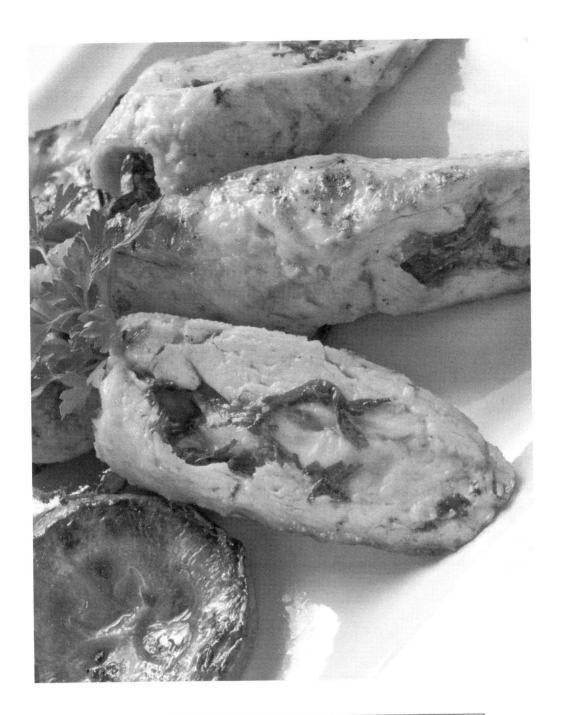

Nutritional Information Per Serving			
Yield:	8 servings	Serving Size:	1 roll
Calories:	271	Fat:	11 grams
Carbohydrates:	0.8 grams	Protein:	39 grams
Fiber	0.1 gram		

Stuffed Chicken Rolls

Talk about the best of all worlds; this recipe has three of my favorite things stuffed inside a chicken breast. It makes eight servings and is the perfect dish to serve guests, because it is both delicious and elegant.

Ingredients:

- 6 chicken breasts, pounded to flatten

- ½ teaspoon salt

- ¼ teaspoon pepper

- ½ teaspoon garlic powder

- 6 tablespoons cream cheese

- 3 slices bacon, cooked and diced

- Fresh spinach leaves

Directions:

1. Preheat the oven to 350 degrees Fahrenheit.

2. Mix the salt, pepper, and garlic powder in a small dish and sprinkle over each breast.

3. Turn the breasts over and spread the cream cheese on the entire surface, leaving a margin at the top and bottom for rolling.

4. Sprinkle the bacon on the cream cheese and lay spinach leaves on top of it all.

5. Take the pointed end of the breast and start rolling up. Secure with a toothpick if necessary.

6. Treat a baking pan with nonstick spray and set each roll inside, spacing them so that they do not touch.

7. Bake for 30 to 40 minutes until done.

Slow-Cooked Chicken Coconut Curry

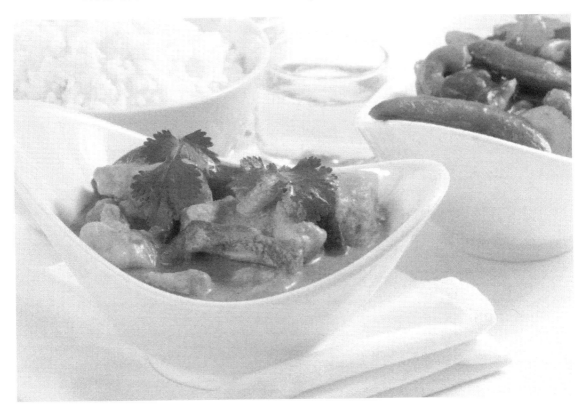

Nutritional Information Per Serving			
Yield:	6 servings	Serving Size:	~1 cup
Calories:	347	Fat:	22 grams
Carbohydrates:	10 grams	Protein:	29 grams
Fiber	4 grams		

Chicken Coconut Curry

This chicken dish contains the exotic flavors of curry and coconut. It also includes fresh pumpkin, but you can always swap out summer squash or butternut squash, if you prefer. I use breasts to make this dish. I'm sure everyone will love it.

Ingredients:

- 1 onion finely sliced

- 1½ cups raw pumpkin, peeled and cubed

- 1¼ cup light coconut milk

- 2 tablespoons curry paste

- 1¾ cup chicken breast, cooked rare and diced

- 1½ cups fresh spinach leaves, chopped

- 3 tablespoons cashews

Directions:

1. Treat the inside of a Crock-Pot with nonstick spray.

2. Place the onion, pumpkin, coconut milk, curry paste, and chicken breast in the Crock-Pot, cover it, and cook for six to 10 hours on low heat or four to six hours on high. Stir occasionally.

3. Ten minutes before you want to serve, add the spinach. It will wilt as it warms. Once it wilts, stir it in.

4. Coconut milk comes in many different textures. If you use one that is very thin, you might need to thicken the mixture before adding the spinach. If necessary, you can use xanthan gum mixed in a little water to thicken it.

5. Serve alone or over riced cauliflower.

Chapter 7: Pork Recipes Fit for Royalty

Pork has always been a favorite in my family. We love pork chops

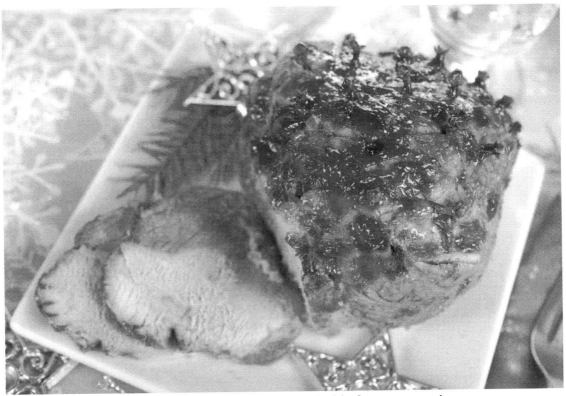

and ham. The following recipes are suitable for any occasion.

Anytime Cranberry-Apricot-Glazed Baked Ham

Nutritional Information Per Serving			
Yield:	18 servings	Serving Size:	4 ounces
Calories:	282	Fat:	19 grams
Carbohydrates:	1 grams	Protein:	24 grams
Fiber	0.4 grams		

Cranberry-Apricot Glazed Ham

This recipe includes my favorite ham glaze probably because I have a sweet tooth and this definitely satisfies. I prefer to use a shank ham with bone in as it is a little sturdier than a boneless ham. This makes 18 servings, so it is suitable for larger groups, but it also freezes well if you want to make it ahead and stash portions in the freezer for later use.

Ingredients:

- 1 10-pound ham with shank

- 2 cups water

- ½ cup water

- 1 cup raw cranberries

- ⅓ cup sugar-free apricot preserves

- 2 tablespoons stevia

- 1 teaspoon ground cardamom

- ½ teaspoon orange zest (Save the orange itself for presentation by slicing thin and twisting.)

Directions:

1. Preheat the oven to 350 degrees Fahrenheit and prepare a roasting pan with non-stick spray. If you have a pan with a rack, use the rack.

2. Score the ham on top and place it in the roasting pan.

3. Pour the two cups of water in the bottom of the pan and bake for one hour.

4. While baking, combine the water, cranberries, and jam in a saucepan on the stove. Bring to a boil and immediately reduce to a simmer for five to seven minutes. The cranberries will burst and the mixture should be thick and bubbly.

5. Use an immersion blender to make it smooth and creamy or pour into a blender, but be careful as this syrupy substance is very hot and can burn your skin.

6. Add the artificial sweetener, cardamom, and orange zest, then blend to smooth.

7. Pour half the sauce into another bowl and set aside.

8. Remove the ham and brush the glaze over the top.

9. Roast for around two and a half more hours, until a meat thermometer reads 140 degrees Fahrenheit.

10. Let the ham rest for 10 to 15 minutes before carving.

11. Decorate your sliced ham with curled orange slices.

12. Warm up the rest of the glaze and serve it in a gravy boat.

Asian Pork Chops

Nutritional Information Per Serving			
Yield:	4 servings	Serving Size:	1 piece
Calories:	211	Fat:	16 grams
Carbohydrates:	12 grams	Protein:	68 grams
Fiber	0 grams		

If you have a desire for Asian flair, then you need to try this chop recipe. It uses lemongrass, sesame oil, fish sauce, and additional flavors from the East. Star anise is a seed pod that appears in the shape of a star. It bears the flavor that is most commonly associated with licorice. The anise star must be ground for this recipe. Use a blender or a mortar and pestle to grind up both the peppercorns and the star anise before using.

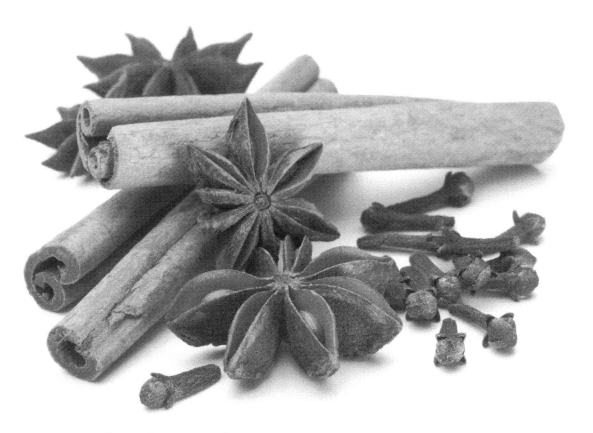

Star anise, grouped with cinnamon sticks and whole cloves

Ingredients:

- 4 boneless pork chops

- 4 garlic cloves, peeled and cut in half, lengthwise

- ¼ teaspoon peppercorns

- 1 medium star anise

- 1 stalk lemongrass, peeled and diced

- 1½ teaspoon coconut aminos

- 1 tablespoon fish sauce

- 1 teaspoon sesame oil

- ½ teaspoon five spice powder

- 1 tablespoon almond flour

- ½ tablespoon sugar-free ketchup (see recipe, Chapter 9)

- ½ tablespoon chili paste

Directions:

1. Pound the pork chops to about ½ inch thick.

2. Peel and halve the garlic cloves and set aside.

3. Grind the peppercorns and star anise to a fine powder and set aside.

4. Peel the lemongrass and garlic and pound on a hard surface to make a puree. Add the peppercorn and star anise powder to the puree in a bowl.

5. Add the coconut aminos, the fish sauce, sesame oil, and five-spice powder, mixing well.

6. Place the chops on a baking dish and pour the lemongrass marinade over the top. Turn to coat both sides of the chop and marinate at room temperature for one to two hours.

7. Heat a skillet on high temperature.

8. Remove the chops from the marinade and coat them with almond flour on both sides.

9. Sear the chops in the skillet on both sides, turning just once and cooking two minutes per side.

10. Transfer the chops to a cutting board and slice into strips.

11. Make a sauce by combining the ketchup and chili paste and serve on the side, along with the strips.

Bacon-Wrapped Pork Roast

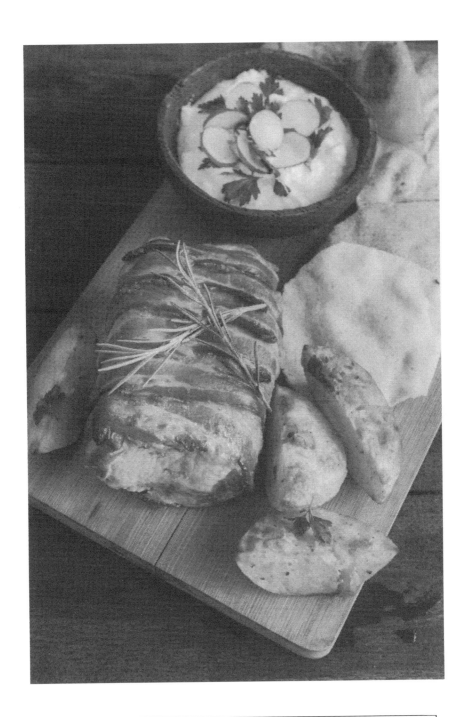

Nutritional Information Per Serving			
Yield:	4 servings	Serving Size:	1 piece
Calories:	605	Fat:	52 grams

Carbohydrates:	3 grams	Protein:	30 grams
Fiber	3 grams		

Bacon-wrapped Pork Roast

Use a pork tenderloin and pound it thin. You'll pile cream cheese, herbs, and the other goodies on top, and then roll it up, covering it with a basket weave of bacon slices. If *that* doesn't make your mouth water, nothing will.

Ingredients:

- 1 16-ounce pork tenderloin

- 1 tablespoon olive oil

- 1 small onion, peeled and sliced

- 2 teaspoons garlic

- 2 ounces fresh spinach

- 3 ounces cream cheese

- ¾ teaspoon dried thyme, divided

- ¾ teaspoon dried rosemary, divided

- ½ teaspoon salt

- ½ teaspoon pepper

- ¾ teaspoon liquid smoke

- 14 slices bacon

Directions:

1. Preheat the oven to 350 degrees Fahrenheit.

2. Prepare the tenderloin by wrapping in plastic wrap and placing on a flat surface. Pound to about three quarters of an inch thick. This takes a while. Massage the meat so that it thins out evenly. Cut off any excess to create a square shape. Set aside.

3. Pour the olive oil into a warmed skillet over high heat and sauté the onions until they are softened.

4. Add the garlic and cook for about one minute, until fragrant.

5. Add the spinach and let it wilt for a minute before adding the cream cheese and stirring it in until it melts.

6. Add a half teaspoon each of thyme and rosemary.

7. Add the salt and pepper and turn to low while you prepare the tenderloin.

8. Make a bacon weave, using the strips of bacon, seven strips across and seven down.

9. Lay the tenderloin on top of the bacon weave and put ¼ teaspoon of the liquid smoke on the surface, reserving the rest for later. Rub the rest of the dried rosemary and thyme on the tenderloin. If any bacon is not even with the tenderloin, trim it flush.

10. With a butter knife, spread the cream cheese and spinach mixture over the tenderloin, leaving a clean margin around the edges.

11. Carefully roll the tenderloin into the bacon and secure it with skewers or toothpicks. You can also tie it with cooking twine, if desired.

12. Bake for 75 minutes in a baking pan prepared with nonstick spray.

13. Let it rest for five minutes, then cut into slices and serve.

Balsamic Roast Tenderloin A La Crock-Pot

Nutritional Information Per Serving			
Yield:	8 servings	Serving Size:	2 burgers
Calories:	188	Fat:	2 grams
Carbohydrates:	1 grams	Protein:	30 grams
Fiber	0 grams		

I love to serve this roast on New Year's Eve, but it is delicious anytime. I am not sure what it is about that balsamic flavor that makes you think of autumn in the air. The vinegar gives it a spicy yet homey flavor. Serve with roasted vegetables from the garden for a tempting treat. Best of all it is made in a Crock-Pot.

Ingredients:

- 1½ tablespoons olive oil

- 4 cloves garlic, peeled and minced

- 1 2-pound pork tenderloin

- 2 tablespoons coconut aminos

- ½ cup balsamic vinegar

- 1 tablespoon Worcestershire sauce

- ½ teaspoon red pepper flakes

- ½ teaspoon sea salt or kosher salt

Directions:

1. Prepare the Crock-Pot by coating the inside with nonstick spray.

2. Pour the olive oil into the bottom of the crock.

3. Sprinkle in the garlic and then set the tenderloin on top.

4. Whisk together the coconut aminos, vinegar, Worcestershire sauce, red pepper flakes, and salt in a bowl; pour over the roast.

5. Set the lid firmly on the Crock-Pot and cook on the high setting for three to four hours or on low for four to six hours.

6. Extract the meat with tongs and place it on a cutting board. Let the meat rest for about five minutes before slicing and arranging the slices on a shallow serving bowl.

7. Pour half of the juice over the meat and place the other half in a gravy boat.

Bourbon-Glazed Ham

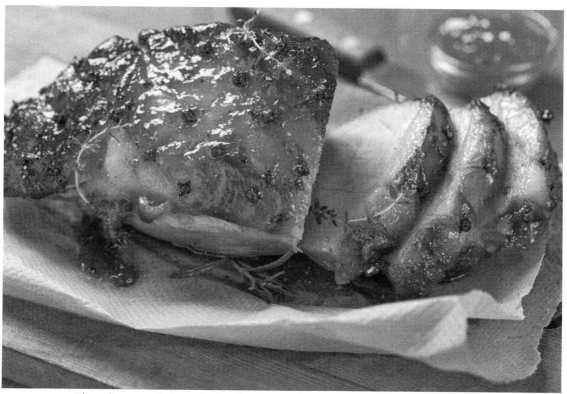

The glaze and the whole cloves up the scrumptious quotient to this ham.

Nutritional Information Per Serving			
Yield:	12 servings	Serving Size:	~2 slices
Calories:	548	Fat:	32 grams
Carbohydrates:	6 grams	Protein:	50 grams
Fiber	0 grams		

Bourbon-Glazed Ham

Here is another glazed ham recipe that is suitable for holidays or anytime. Trust me, you will love this one. It has a spicy, earthy, yet sweet flavor that only a bourbon glaze can impart. I found that the best artificial sweetener to use in this recipe is stevia. Other sweeteners just don't stand up to the alcohol.

Ingredients:

- 1 10- to 12-pound ham with shank in

- Whole cloves

- 1¼ cup stevia

- 1 teaspoon ground mustard

- 1 teaspoon champagne vinegar

- 2 ounces bourbon

Directions:

1. Preheat the oven to 325 degrees and prepare a roasting pan by coating it with nonstick spray.

2. Prepare the ham by scoring the top and inserting cloves in the center of each diamond.

3. Place the ham in the pan and pour in two inches of water. Cover and cook for one hour.

4. Meanwhile, prepare the glaze in a medium saucepan. Combine the stevia, mustard, vinegar, and bourbon. Bring to a slight boil, stirring constantly, then turn off the heat.

5. Remove the ham from the oven and drain off most of the water, if there is any. Apply the glaze to the top of the ham and place back in the oven to cook another hour uncovered.

6. Let the ham rest about 10 minutes before slicing and serving.

Holiday-Worthy Crispy Roast Pork Leg

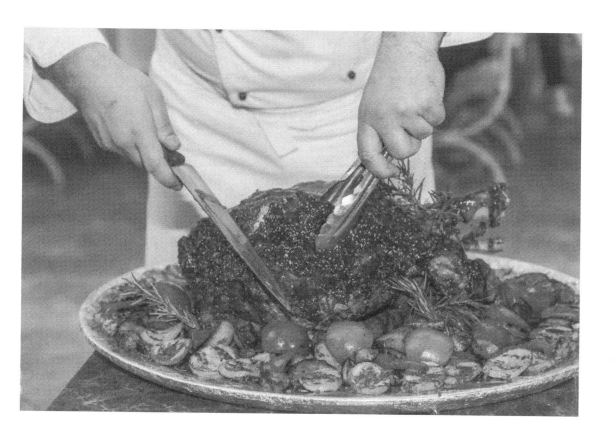

Nutritional Information Per Serving			
Yield:	12 servings	Serving Size:	2 slices
Calories:	252	Fat:	7 grams
Carbohydrates:	3 grams	Protein:	43 grams
Fiber	0.6 grams		

Crispy Roast Pork Leg

That crispy crackling that forms on a leg of pork is beyond delicious. You can achieve that with this recipe that fits right in with your low-carb diet. I like to serve this around Christmas, along with ham because it does taste differently delicious. The recipe is large enough that you can feed a crowd.

Ingredients:

- 1 4-pound pork leg

161

- 2 tablespoons olive oil

- 1 tablespoon garlic powder

- 1 tablespoon dried rosemary

- 1½ teaspoons salt

- 1 medium onion, peeled and sliced

- 1 cup mushrooms, sliced

- 1 teaspoon fennel seed

- 4 cloves of garlic, peeled

Directions:

1. Preheat the oven to 425 degrees Fahrenheit.

2. Prepare a roasting pan by lining it with foil and coating this with nonstick spray.

3. Rinse the pork leg and pat it dry with a paper towel.

4. Rub the leg with the olive oil.

5. In a small bowl, whisk together the garlic powder, rosemary, and salt. Rub this on the pork leg.

6. Place the sliced onion and mushrooms in the roasting pan. Set the pork leg on top.

7. Sprinkle the fennel seed and garlic cloves on top.

8. Cover lightly with foil and place in the oven for 45 to 50 minutes.

9. Lower the oven temperature to 350 degrees Fahrenheit and cook the roast, uncovered, for 90 more minutes.

10. Remove from the oven and let the leg rest for 10 minutes before slicing.

Parmesan Pork Chops

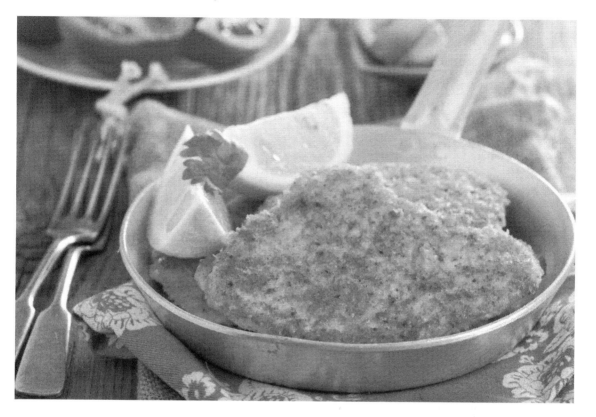

Nutritional Information Per Serving			
Yield:	4 servings	Serving Size:	2 chops
Calories:	509	Fat:	32 grams
Carbohydrates:	4 grams	Protein:	52 grams
Fiber	0 grams		

Parmesan Pork Chops

I love these chops because they come out crispy and delicious. The Parmesan cheese makes a nice crust and gives a solid crunch when you bite into one. This recipe makes eight pork chops; I suggest using a thin center-cut boneless chop.

Ingredients:

- 2 tablespoons butter, melted

- 2 tablespoons coconut oil, melted

- 4 cloves garlic, peeled and minced

- 1 teaspoon dried thyme

- 1 tablespoon dried parsley

- ¼ teaspoon sea salt

- ¼ teaspoon cracked pepper

- ¾ cup Parmesan cheese, grated

- 8 center-cut pork chops

Directions:

1. Preheat the oven to 400 degrees Fahrenheit and cover a baking pan with parchment paper. Coat the parchment paper with nonstick spray and set the pan aside.

2. Melt the butter and coconut oil together and pour into a bowl.

3. Add the garlic, thyme, parsley, salt, pepper, and Parmesan cheese; mix well.

4. Place the chops on the baking sheet and divide the spice and butter mixture on top of each, spreading it over the chops.

5. Bake for 20 to 25 minutes or until the chops are done. Check with a meat thermometer for 135 degrees Fahrenheit.

6. If any of the butter mixture has gathered on the pan, spoon it on top of the chops when serving.

Pork And Veggie Stir Fry

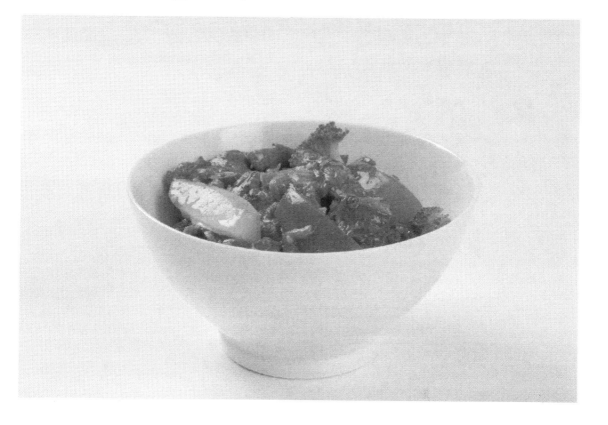

Nutritional Information Per Serving			
Yield:	4 servings	Serving Size:	~1 cup
Calories:	226	Fat:	12 grams
Carbohydrates:	10 grams	Protein:	19 grams
Fiber	1 gram		

Pork and Veggie Stir Fry

Pork is used in lots of stir fry recipes; it makes for a delicious low-carb dinner that is ready in a flash. The vegetables are placed in a bowl in a specific succession so the items that take the longest to cook are added first and will be fully cooked when those that needs less time are done. I prefer to cut the pork into strips, because it is easier to eat with chopsticks. If you would rather cut them in cubes you may, but they will take a little longer to cook.

Ingredients:

- 1 teaspoon garlic, peeled and minced

- 1 tablespoon fresh ginger, peeled and minced

- ¾ pound pork loin, cut in thin strips or cubes

- 2 tablespoons olive oil, divided

- 1 red bell pepper, seeded and sliced into thin strips

- ½ cup green onions, cleaned and sliced thin

- 1 cup fresh broccoli florets

- 1 tablespoon stevia

- 1 teaspoon arrowroot powder

- 2 tablespoons coconut aminos

- 1 tablespoon dry sherry

- 1 teaspoon sesame oil

Directions:

1. Mix the garlic and ginger together well.

2. Slice the pork into thin strips and toss it with one tablespoon of olive oil and the garlic/ginger mixture. Set aside.

3. Place the strips of bell pepper in the bottom of a medium bowl and top with the green onions. Layer the broccoli florets on the top. Set aside.

4. In a small bowl combine with the arrowroot powder. Stir in the coconut aminos, the sherry, and the sesame oil and mix well. Set aside.

5. Place the wok over high heat. It must be very hot. To test it, drop a bit of water on the wok; when it skips across the surface, the wok is ready.

6. Add the additional tablespoon of olive oil and tilt the wok to coat it. Pour out any remaining oil. Add the pork mixture to the wok and stir quickly to brown it on all sides in the bottom of the pan. Leave it in the bottom, without stirring until the meat turns white but it is not cooked all the way through. Stir again until it is almost cooked through. Remove to a serving dish.

7. Dump the vegetable bowl in the wok so that the broccoli is on the bottom. Cover the wok with a lid and let the contents cook for one minute. Remove the lid and stir the vegetables.

8. Dump the pork and any juices back into the wok and stir fry for a minute or two.

9. Add the sauce over the pork and vegetables and push everything to the side while the sauce starts to boil in the bottom. Stir the sauce occasionally until it starts to thicken.

10. Mix everything together once it thickens and serve immediately.

Pork Chops With Velvety Gravy

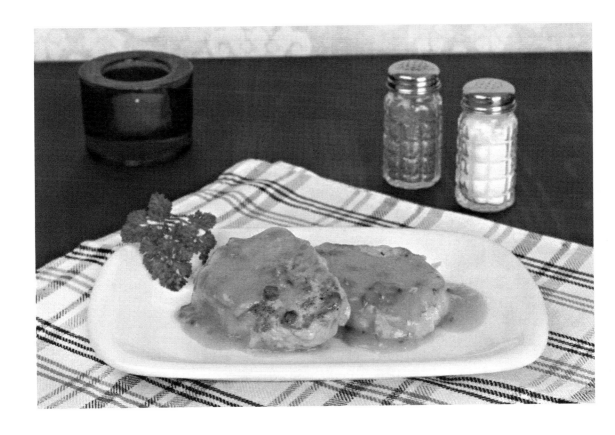

Nutritional Information Per Serving			
Yield:	4 servings	Serving Size:	1 chop
Calories:	305	Fat:	18 grams
Carbohydrates:	6 grams	Protein:	37 grams
Fiber	1 gram		

Pork Chops With Velvety Gravy

Pork chops are a comfort food for me. My mom made the best smothered chops with gravy ever and served them with mashed potatoes. Now I switch out those potatoes for mashed cauliflower or a carrot puree for a delicious meal.

Ingredients:

- 6 slices bacon

- 1 medium onion, peeled and sliced thin

- ¼ teaspoon salt

- ⅛ teaspoon pepper

- 4 pork chops, about one inch thick with bone in

- ½ cup chicken broth

- ¼ cup heavy cream

Directions:

1. In a large skillet, cook the bacon until crisp. Remove to a paper towel to drain and reserve the grease.

2. Add the onions in the pan with the grease and sauté over low heat. Add salt and pepper and stir, cooking until the onions are golden brown.

3. Crumble the bacon and place in a heatproof bowl. Remove the onions with a slotted spoon and add them to the bacon.

4. Sprinkle the chops with a little salt and pepper and place them the skillet, turning the heat up to medium high. Brown on one side for three minutes then turn, reduce heat to medium, and cook for 10 minutes. Check with a meat thermometer to ensure the chops are 135 degrees Fahrenheit.

5. Remove the meat to a platter and cover with foil to keep warm.

6. Pour the chicken broth and cream into the skillet. Bring to a simmer and stir, scraping the brown bits into the gravy. The mixture should thicken after two to three minutes. Add the bacon and onions and combine. Serve, topping the chops with gravy.

Pulled Pork

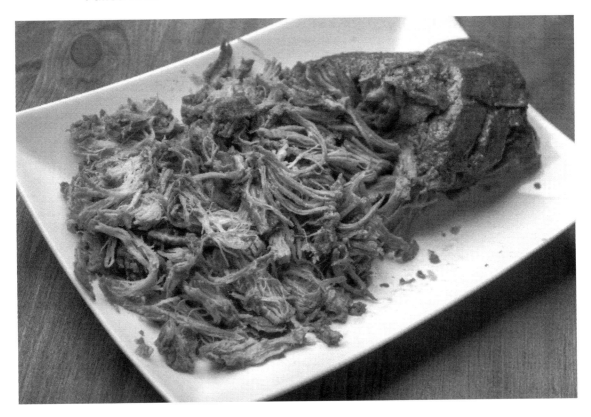

Nutritional Information Per Serving			
Yield:	24 servings	Serving Size:	6 ounces
Calories:	315	Fat:	21 grams
Carbohydrates:	0.5 gram	Protein:	30 grams
Fiber	0 grams		

Pulled Pork

I never liked my pulled pork in a bun anyway. I now spoon some onto a leaf of romaine lettuce, fold it up, and eat it like a lettuce wrap. I love the spicy flavor of the pork and the lettuce leaf adds crunch, if you eat it right away. You must brine the pork overnight and it takes about three hours to cook just the pork butt, so this takes a little time to prepare. It is very worth the effort, though.

Ingredients

Brine:

- 1 9-pound pork butt

- ½ cup salt

- 2 tablespoons liquid smoke

- Water

Rub:

- 2 teaspoons paprika

- 1½ teaspoon cayenne pepper

- 3 teaspoons salt

- 4 teaspoons ground black pepper

- ¼ cup prepared mustard

- 2 teaspoons liquid smoke

Directions:

1. Cut the pork butt in half.

2. Place the pieces of pork butt in a large pot and pour in the salt and liquid smoke. Fill with enough water to cover the meat.

3. Leave the pork butt in the brine for at least 90 minutes, preferably overnight.

4. In a bowl, combine the paprika, cayenne pepper, salt, and black pepper.

5. Remove the meat from the brine and pat it dry with paper towels.

6. Rub the dry mixture all over the surface of the meat.

7. In another bowl, combine the mustard and liquid smoke. Add this to the surface of the meat.

8. Place the meat in a large baking dish, wrapping it first with parchment paper and then aluminum foil.

9. Bake in a preheated 325-degree Fahrenheit oven for three hours.

10. Remove from the oven and unwrap.

11. Turn the oven to 375 degrees Fahrenheit and bake the meat, uncovered, for another 90 minutes, or until the internal temperature, is 190 degrees.

12. Let the meat cool for a few minutes before shredding with two forks.

13. Serve with your favorite keto barbeque sauce.

Chapter 8: Tender and Tasty Low-Carb Lamb

Lamb is something most of us Americans ignore. Lamb is a major meat group in other countries and therefore, some of the recipes in this book come from outside of the US. Lamb is a great source of protein, making it perfect for a ketogenic diet.

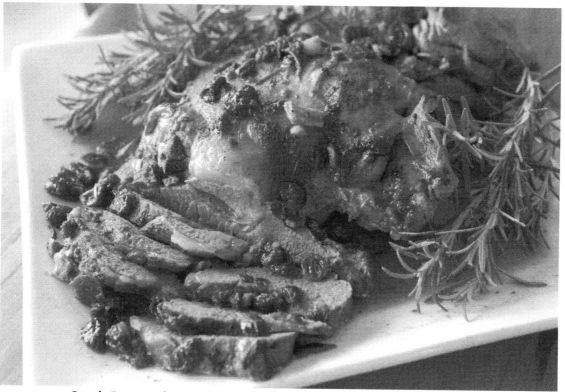

Crock-Pot Lamb Roast

Nutritional Information Per Serving			
Yield:	6 servings	Serving Size:	~4 slices
Calories:	414	Fat:	35 grams
Carbohydrates:	0.5 gram	Protein:	27 grams
Fiber	0 grams		

Lamb Roast

I sometimes have a hard time getting lamb roast to come out the way I want it to. It can become tough and stringy very easily. Because this recipe is made in a Crock-Pot, you will not have that problem. The meat will be so tender it will fall apart and melt in your mouth.

Ingredients:

- 1 2-pound leg of lamb
- 2 cloves garlic, peeled and cut into three pieces each
- ¼ teaspoon dried rosemary
- ¼ cup olive oil
- 2 tablespoons grainy brown mustard
- 1 tablespoon maple syrup (use real maple syrup)
- Salt and pepper to taste
- 4 sprigs thyme
- 6 fresh mint leaves
- salt and pepper to taste

Directions:

1. Make three large slits on the top of the leg of lamb, about 1½-inches deep.

2. Using your fingers, insert two pieces of garlic and some of the rosemary in each of these slits and pinch the slits together.

3. In a small bowl, combine the olive oil, mustard, maple syrup, salt, and pepper. Rub this all over the leg of lamb and place it in the Crock-Pot.

4. Put the lid on the Crock-Pot and cook the meat for seven hours on low heat. Once the juices start gathering around the lamb (about six hours), add the sprigs of thyme and mint leaves, and continue to cook.

5. Remove the lamb and let it set for 10 minutes before slicing and serving.

Exotic Lamb Curry With Spinach (Saag Gosht)

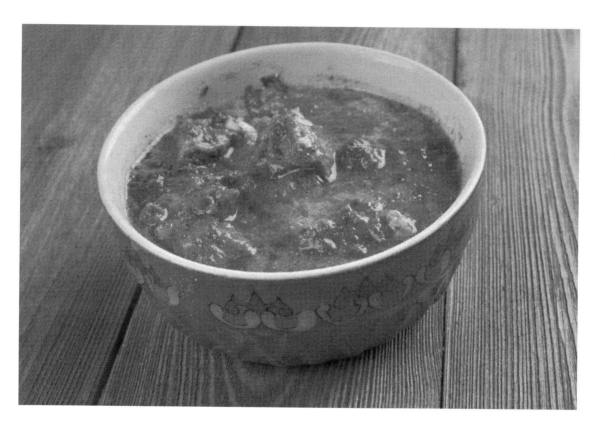

Nutritional Information Per Serving			
Yield:	6 servings	Serving Size:	~1 cup
Calories:	158	Fat:	6 grams
Carbohydrates:	8 grams	Protein:	20 grams
Fiber	0.8 gram		

Saag Gosht

This recipe is also cooked in a Crock-pot; it brings a little of the Near East to our dinner table. It calls for spices like ginger, cardamom, and whole cloves, along with turmeric, chili powder, garam masala powder, and cumin.

This recipe comes from Northern India and definitely has an exotic flavor. I serve it over riced cauliflower and my family devours it in seconds. I'm sure yours will, too. It provides a pleasant change from normal, everyday fare.

Note: the provided nutritional information does not include the riced cauliflower. You can find this information in Chapter 9 under the name "Faux Rice."

Ingredients:

- 1½-pound lamb, cubed

- Salt and pepper to taste

- 1 tablespoon olive oil

- 1 16-ounce bag frozen spinach

- 1 red onion, peeled and sliced

- 2 cloves garlic, peeled and crushed

- 1 tablespoon fresh ginger, crushed

- 2 teaspoons coriander

- 1 teaspoon turmeric powder

- ½ teaspoon chili powder

- 1 teaspoon garam masala powder

- 1 28-ounce can crushed tomatoes

Directions:

1. Season the lamb cubes with salt and pepper to taste.

2. Add the olive oil to a hot skillet and brown the lamb cubes on all sides.

3. Place the lamb into the bottom of a crock pot.

4. Defrost and drain the spinach. Squeeze out as much liquid as you can.

5. Place the spinach in the Crock-Pot along with the onion, garlic, ginger, coriander, turmeric, chili powder, garam masala powder, and the crushed tomatoes. Stir all the ingredients together.

6. Set the lid on the Crock-Pot and cook on the high setting for four to five hours or on low for eight hours.

Greek Lamb Burgers With Mint

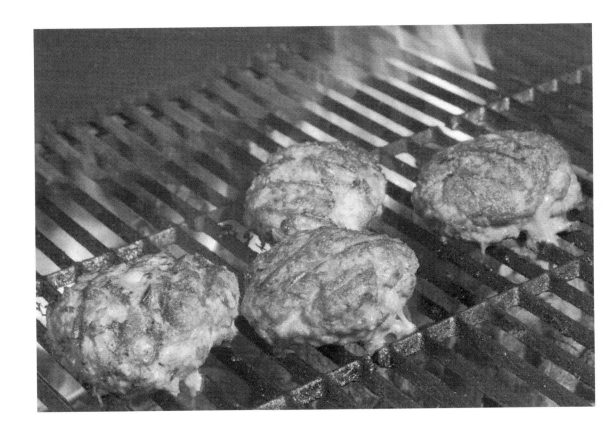

Nutritional Information Per Serving			
Yield:	4 servings	Serving Size:	1 burger
Calories:	300	Fat:	20 grams
Carbohydrates:	3 grams	Protein:	25 grams
Fiber	2 grams		

Greek Lamb Burgers

The addition of a little feta cheese to the burgers before serving them only adds to their pizzazz.

Ingredients:

- 1-pound ground lamb

- ½ cup fresh mint, chopped

- 3 tablespoons rosemary

- Salt and pepper to taste

- 1 tablespoon olive oil

- 2 tablespoons feta cheese

Directions:

1. Place the lamb in a bowl and break it apart with a fork or a large spoon.

2. Add the mint, rosemary, salt, and pepper to the bowl and mix with your hands.

3. Form into four burger shapes and firmly squish each piece together.

4. Heat a skillet over medium high heat and pour in the olive oil. Brown each side of the burgers, cooking about five to eight minutes per side.

Italian Lamb Chops With Fresh Pesto

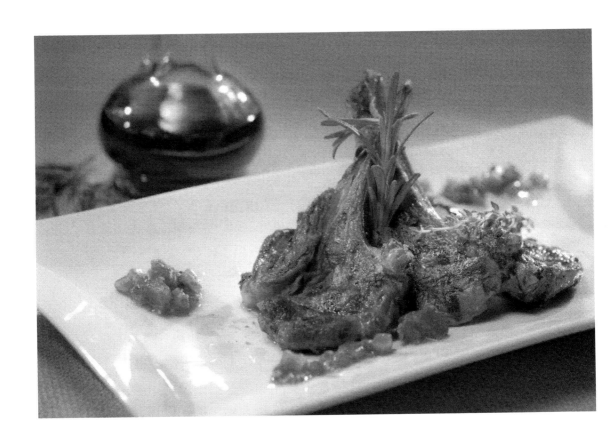

Nutritional Information Per Serving			
Yield:	4 servings	Serving Size:	2 chops
Calories:	603	Fat:	51 grams
Carbohydrates:	3 grams	Protein:	35 grams
Fiber	1 gram		

Italian Lamb Chops with Pesto

Pesto is one of my favorite things, so I was thrilled to be able to present this recipe. The pesto is a great enhancement to the meat.

Ingredients:

- 2 tablespoons ghee

- 1 rack of lamb

- Sea salt and ground pepper to taste

- 4 cups fresh basil leaves

- ¼ teaspoon sea salt

- ⅛ teaspoon ground pepper

- ½ cup pine nuts

- ½ cup olive oil

- Juice of one lemon

Directions:

1. Preheat the oven to 350 degrees Fahrenheit.

2. Use a large oven-safe skillet and place it on the stove over medium high heat.

3. Melt the ghee in the skillet.

4. Sprinkle the rack of lamb with sea salt and ground pepper.

5. When the skillet becomes hot, set the meat on one side, pressing down slightly to help it sear. Rotate the meat until all sides are seared.

6. Set the skillet in the oven for 10 minutes for a medium finish, 11-12 minutes for well done.

7. Remove from the oven and place the lamb on a cutting board. Let it rest until the pesto is ready.

8. Put the basil, salt, pepper, pine nuts, olive oil, and lemon juice in a food processor and pulse until creamy, scraping down the sides as needed. If the consistency becomes too thick, feel free to add a little more oil.

9. Slice the rack of lamb into chops and arrange on four plates. Top with pesto and serve.

Moroccan Lamb Chops

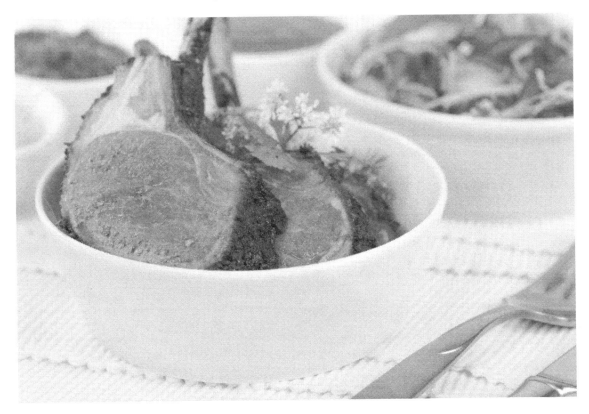

Nutritional Information Per Serving			
Yield:	4 servings	Serving Size:	2 chops
Calories:	519	Fat:	43 grams
Carbohydrates:	2 grams	Protein:	31 grams
Fiber	0 grams		

Moroccan Lamb Chops

In this recipe, you grill the lamb chops; they just don't taste right if you cook them on the stove. You'll also be making a chermoula sauce that is simultaneously spicy and minty.

Ingredients:

- 2 tablespoons fresh mint, chopped
- ¼ cup fresh parsley, chopped
- 3 cloves garlic, peeled and chopped
- 2 tablespoons lemon zest
- ½ teaspoon smoked paprika
- 1 teaspoon red pepper flakes
- 2 tablespoons lemon juice
- ¼ cup olive oil
- salt and pepper to taste
- ¾ teaspoon salt
- ¾ teaspoon pepper
- ¼ teaspoon cumin
- 1 teaspoon olive oil
- 8 lamb loin chops

Directions:

1. Make the chermoula sauce by combining the mint, parsley, garlic, lemon zest, paprika, pepper flakes, lemon juice, salt, and pepper to taste in a blender. The mixture should be thick and not totally liquid. It should look like pesto. Set aside.

2. In a small bowl combine ¾ teaspoon salt, ¾ teaspoon pepper, and the cumin, mixing well.

183

3. Coat the lamb chops with the olive oil and rub the entire surface with the cumin mixture.

4. Grill for about two minutes on each side for medium rare and about three minutes if you like your chops more well-done.

5. Serve the chops, topped with a couple tablespoons of chermoula sauce, each.

Not-So-Irish Lamb Stew

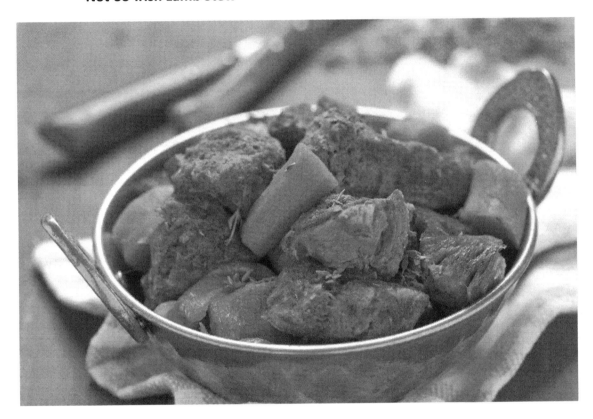

Nutritional Information Per Serving			
Yield:	4 servings	Serving Size:	1 bowl
Calories:	782	Fat:	45 grams
Carbohydrates:	13 grams	Protein:	72 grams
Fiber	0.4 grams		

Not-so-Irish Lamb Stew

I grew up on lamb stew and, honestly, I did not like it much. I don't think grandma actually used lamb, but probably mutton. Mutton is an older sheep while lamb comes from sheep under three years of age. Mutton is a stronger flavor and it is also tougher. When I actually had lamb stew with real lamb, I found I liked it. This stew is very garlicky; in fact, you use a whole bulb of garlic. This recipe uses the stove in a Dutch oven, but you can just as easily cook it in a Crock-Pot.

Ingredients:

- 1 2-pound leg of lamb

- 2 tablespoons olive oil

- Salt and pepper to taste

- 1 onion, peeled and sliced

- 3 carrots, peeled and chopped

- 1 bulb garlic, each clove peeled and crushed

- 1 tomato, chopped

- 2 tablespoons butter

- 1 cup beef broth

- 1 cup white wine

- 2 sprigs rosemary

- 1 teaspoon dried thyme

- ½ teaspoon salt

- ¼ teaspoon pepper

Directions:

1. Place the Dutch oven on the stove over high heat until it gets hot. While warming, rub the leg of lamb with olive oil and season it with salt and pepper.

2. Brown the leg of lamb on all sides. Remove from Dutch oven and set on a plate.

3. Place the onions and carrots in the Dutch oven and sauté until the onions become translucent.

4. Add the garlic and tomato, stirring to mix well.

5. Pour in the beef broth and the white wine, then toss in the rosemary, thyme, salt, and pepper.

6. Immerse the leg of lamb in the liquid and bring it to a boil. Reduce the heat to a low simmer and let it cook for about four hours.

7. The leg should be fork tender by this time. Remove the lamb from the bone and stir everything together. Serve in bowls.

Pan-Seared Lamb Chops In Mustard Sauce

Nutritional Information Per Serving			
Yield:	4 servings	Serving Size:	2 chops
Calories:	426	Fat:	30 grams
Carbohydrates:	4 grams	Protein:	31 grams
Fiber	0 grams		

If you like mustard, you will love this recipe. The creamy sauce is spicy and sweet. The best thing about this recipe is it takes only about a half hour to make and have on the table, but you do have to prep and marinate the chops the day before.

Ingredients:

- 2 cloves garlic, peeled and minced
- 1 tablespoons fresh rosemary, minced
- 1 tablespoons olive oil
- 8 lamb chops, trimmed
- Salt and pepper to taste
- 1 tablespoon green onion, chopped
- 1 more tablespoon olive oil
- ½ cup unsalted beef broth
- 2 tablespoons brandy
- 1 tablespoon grainy brown mustard, prepared
- 2 teaspoons Worcestershire sauce
- 1 teaspoon powdered artificial sweetener
- ⅔ cup heavy cream
- 1 sprig of thyme
- 1 sprig of rosemary
- 2 teaspoons fresh lemon juice
- 2 tablespoons butter

Directions:

1. The day before, mix the garlic and rosemary in a small bowl and add one tablespoon of olive oil. Mix well.

2. Trim all but ⅛ inch of fat off the lamb chops. Set the chops in the bottom of a baking dish and season with salt and pepper. Smear a bit of the garlic mixture on each side of each chop. Cover with plastic wrap and place in the refrigerator overnight.

3. To cook, bring the chops to room temperature by letting them set out for 30 minutes.

4. Heat a large nonstick or stainless skillet over medium high heat, then add the other tablespoon of olive oil, coating the bottom of the pan. Add as many lamb chops as you can to make a single layer in the skillet and turn the heat down to medium. Cook undisturbed for six minutes before turning and cooking another six minutes. If you like your chops well-done, leave them in another minute on both sides.

5. Take the chops out and place on a plate covering loosely with foil.

6. In the same skillet, bring the heat to medium low, add the green onions, and sauté until soft.

7. Add both broth and brandy and simmer for one minute. Add the mustard, Worcestershire sauce, and sweetener. Whisk well.

8. Add the cream and whisk together thoroughly. As the mixture heats up, add the sprigs of thyme and rosemary then simmer for eight minutes.

9. Add the lemon juice mixture along with the butter and stir until the sauce becomes glossy and thickens. It will thicken even more as it cools.

10. Remove the rosemary and thyme sprigs before spooning the sauce over the lamb chops.

Roast Leg Of Lamb

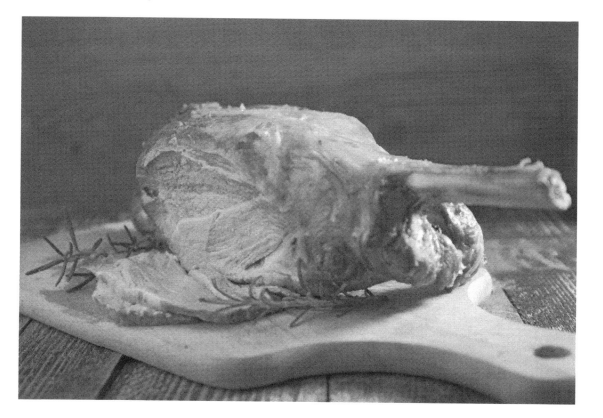

Nutritional Information Per Serving			
Yield:	6 servings	Serving Size:	¼ ounce
Calories:	594	Fat:	44 grams
Carbohydrates:	3 grams	Protein:	40 grams
Fiber	0 grams		

Roast Leg of Lamb

Leg of lamb is a great dish to serve when guests come over. It fills the house with a wonderful fragrance and isn't as hard to cook as you might imagine. Lamb is very fatty; that's what gives it such a wonderful flavor. Once you try roast lamb, it will become a favorite.

Ingredients:

- 1 3-pound boneless leg of lamb
- 2 tablespoons garlic, peeled and minced
- 1 teaspoon dried thyme
- 1 teaspoon dried rosemary
- ½ teaspoon salt
- ¼ teaspoon pepper
- 1 tablespoon lemon juice
- 1 tablespoon olive oil
- ½ cup dry red wine
- 2 tablespoons butter
- Twine

Directions:

1. Preheat the oven to 450 degrees Fahrenheit.

2. Trim all but about a quarter to a half inch of the fat off the fatty side of the lamb. Score the fat with a crisscross pattern.

3. In a bowl, mix the garlic, thyme, rosemary, salt, pepper, lemon juice, and olive oil to form a thin paste. Apply this to both sides of the lamb.

4. Use the twine to truss the leg closed.

5. Place in a nonstick sprayed roasting pan and cook for 15 minutes.

6. Reduce the oven heat to 325 degrees Fahrenheit and cook for 45 more minutes. Check, using a meat thermometer. For medium rare, the internal temperature should be 135 degrees. Cook a little longer for medium.

7. Let the roast rest at least five minutes before removing the twine.

8. Add the wine to the roasting pan to deglaze it. Remove the wine and drippings to a small saucepan and add the butter. Simmer until reduced by half.

9. Slice the meat and serve with au jus.

Tender Lamb Shanks À La Crock Pot

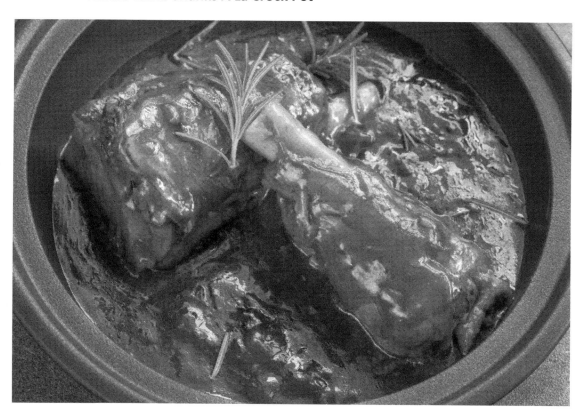

Nutritional Information Per Serving

Yield:	6 servings	Serving Size:	1 piece
Calories:	762	Fat:	31 grams
Carbohydrates:	11 grams	Protein:	58 grams
Fiber	2 grams		

Lamb Shanks

Slow-cooking the lamb shanks makes them tender and delicious. The sauce is incredible in this dish and is delicious served over riced cauliflower (nutrients not included in the total nutritional information, above).

Ingredients:

- 6 lamb shanks

- 1 teaspoon salt

- 1 teaspoon pepper

- 1 tablespoon olive oil

- 2 carrots, peeled and chopped

- 2 stalks celery, chopped

- 1 onion, peeled and chopped

- 1 tablespoon dried oregano

- 2 tablespoons dried rosemary

- 1 28-ounce can crushed tomatoes

- 1 cup red wine

- 1½ cups chicken stock

- 3 bay leaves

Directions:

1. Heat olive oil in a large skillet over medium heat. Season lamb shanks with salt and pepper and put them in the skillet to brown on all sides. Do not cook the meat, just brown them. Remove the meat to a plate and set aside.

2. In the same skillet, sauté the carrot, celery, and onion until soft, about five minutes.

3. Add the oregano and rosemary and stir for about two minutes.

4. Add the tomatoes, wine, and chicken stock and stir well. Simmer for five minutes.

5. Place the lamb shanks in the Crock-Pot on top of the vegetables.

6. Pour the sauce into the Crock-Pot on top of the lamb shanks.

7. Add the bay leaves.

8. Cook on low for eight hours.

Turkish Lamb With Low-Carb Pita

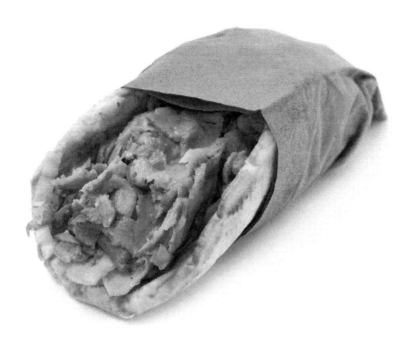

Nutritional Information Per Serving			
Yield:	4 servings	Serving Size:	1 full pita
Calories:	730	Fat:	45 grams
Carbohydrates:	9 grams	Protein:	60 grams
Fiber	11 grams		

Turkish Lamb with Low-carb Pita

Pita does have carbs, so it is necessary to make a low-carb pita with which to serve this dish. A trip to your local grocery and health food store should give you everything you need, including ground flaxseed, ground chia seeds, coconut flour, a head of cauliflower, and some eggs. You serve the lamb in the low-carb pita bread along with vegetables and some fresh tasting ingredients.

Ingredients:

Pita:

- ½ small head of cauliflower

- 1 tablespoon water

- ¼ cup ground flaxseed

- ¼ cup ground chia seed

- 2½ tablespoon coconut flour

- 1 teaspoon baking soda

- 2 medium eggs

- ¼ cup olive oil

Lamb:

- Salt and pepper to taste

- 1½-pound ground lamb

- 1 small red onion, peeled and chopped

- 2 cloves garlic, peeled and minced

- 1 teaspoon cinnamon

- 2 teaspoons ground cumin

- 2 teaspoons paprika

- 1 tablespoon tomato paste

- 1 cup chicken stock

- 1 bunch fresh mint leaves

- 4 tablespoons pomegranate seeds

- 2 tablespoons pine nuts

- ½ cup fresh feta cheese

- 2 tablespoons fresh parsley

Directions:

Pita:

1. Preheat oven to 375 degrees Fahrenheit.

2. Chop the cauliflower into chunks and put in food processor to process at high speed with a five blade or grating blade. You want it to look like rice when it is done. Put the cauliflower in a microwave safe bowl with one tablespoon water and cook on high in microwave for four to five minutes.

3. Pour cauliflower in a muslin bag and squeeze out all excess water.

4. If you can't get ground flax or chia seeds, whirl them in the blender at high speed for 10 seconds. Whisk the ground seeds with baking soda, coconut flour and add the cauliflower and coat well.

5. In a deep bowl, crack the eggs. Add the olive oil and whisk. Add the flaxseed mixture to the wet mixture. Stand for two minutes to thicken.

6. Line a baking pan with parchment paper and divide dough in four parts and spoon onto the parchment. Flatten with a spatula to about ½ inch thick and put in the oven for 18 minutes.

Lamb:

7. Meanwhile, put a Dutch oven on the stove and warm it over medium high heat. Add the lamb and brown for about 10 minutes.

8. Add the onion and the garlic and cook five to six more minutes.

9. Add the cinnamon, cumin, paprika, tomato paste, salt, and pepper and cook for one more minute.

10. Add the chicken stock and bring to a boil. Turn the heat to low and simmer for eight minutes. The liquid should absorb completely.

11. Add the mint leaves and half of the parsley and mix well. The rest of the parsley will be used for garnish.

12. Place one of the cauliflower pitas on a plate and top with the lamb mixture. Garnish with pomegranate seeds, pine nuts, feta cheese, and parsley.

The next chapter will give you a variety of seafood options to enjoy.

Chapter 9: Melt In Your Mouth Seafood Dishes

Seafood is a high-protein source that is low in cholesterol. The vitamins and minerals that come from seafood are rich in omega-3 fatty acids. It is a good thing to include seafood in a low-carb diet because of these minerals and vitamins, as well as to give your diet additional diversity.

Bacon And Shrimp

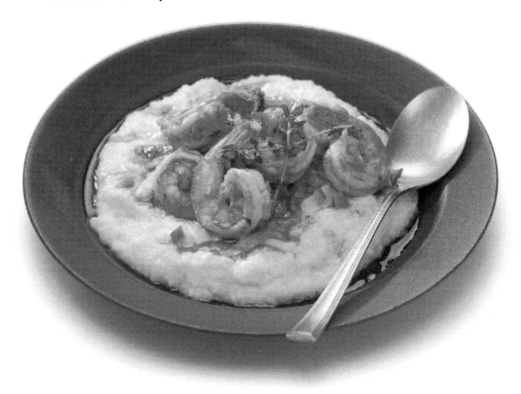

Bacon and shrimp, served on a bed of mashed cauliflower.

Nutritional Information Per Serving			
Yield:	2 servings	Serving Size:	½ total
Calories:	430	Fat:	25 grams

Carbohydrates:	1 grams	Protein:	50 grams
Fiber	0 grams		

Bacon and Shrimp

Here's an easy shrimp recipe that you can have on the table in a flash. You can even cook up your bacon ahead of time. Always use unsalted butter or your dish will be very salty. I often serve this dish with zucchini noodles or cauliflower rice.

Ingredients:

- 8 slices of bacon

- 2 tablespoons unsalted butter

- 12 ounces shrimp, deveined and peeled

- Fresh parsley

Directions:

1. Cut the bacon strips into 1-inch pieces.

2. Melt the butter in a large frying pan and add the bacon frying until crispy.

3. Add the shrimp and cook each side three to four minutes or until they are cooked through.

4. Remove from the heat and serve with fresh, chopped parsley.

Cauliflower Fish Cakes With Aioli

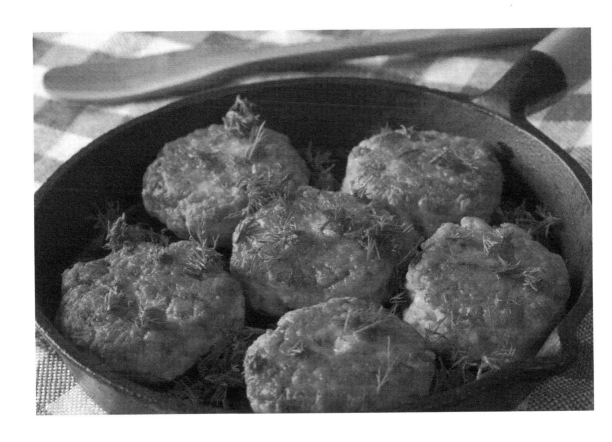

Nutritional Information Per Serving			
Yield:	6 servings	Serving Size:	3 cakes
Calories:	449	Fat:	34 grams
Carbohydrates:	6 grams	Protein:	30 grams
Fiber	3 grams		

Cauliflower Fish Cakes with Aioli

My mother used to make fish cakes as a way of stretching a meal, but what was in it was not particularly good for a low-carb diet. This recipe stretches that food dollar without adding breading to the mix. Instead of bread, rice, or flour, you use cauliflower rice (see Chapter 9 for instructions). It is served with an aioli, a flavored mayonnaise that works like tartar sauce. This recipe makes 18 fish cakes.

Ingredients:

- 2 cups cauliflower rice

- 4 tablespoons ghee, divided

- 1 clove garlic, peeled and minced

- 2 pounds white fish fillets (haddock or cod)

- ½ teaspoon salt

- ½ teaspoon ground pepper

- 1 teaspoon lemon zest

- 2 tablespoons fresh parsley

- 1 teaspoon ground cumin

- 2 green onions, chopped

- 2 large eggs

- ½ cup grated Parmesan cheese

- 4 tablespoons flax meal

- ½ cup mayonnaise (see the recipe in the next chapter)

- 2 cloves garlic, peeled and minced

Directions:

1. Place one tablespoon of the ghee in a skillet over medium heat and add the garlic. Sauté about 30 seconds and add the cauliflower rice. Season with a little salt and cook while stirring for five to seven minutes. Take off the stove and set aside.

2. Pat the fish fillets dry with a paper towel and season with salt and pepper.

3. Set a large skillet over medium heat and add another tablespoon of ghee. Add the fish and cook for two to three minutes, flip and cook another two to three minutes. When done, the fillet should be opaque and will flake easily.

4. Put the cauliflower rice in a bowl along with the fish fillets and add lemon zest, parsley, cumin, onion, eggs, Parmesan cheese, and flax meal. Season with salt and pepper and mix well with a fork, or your hands.

5. Use a ¼ cup measuring cup as a mold, spooning the fish mixture in and pressing it down. Turn it out on a cutting board and use your hands to shape the contents into a patty.

6. Heat another tablespoon of ghee in a clean skillet over medium high heat. Once it is hot, reduce to medium heat, and introduce the fish patties. Cook these for three to five minutes on each side or until golden brown. Don't flip these patties too early or the crust will break and the fish will go everywhere. Work in batches of four to five cakes at a time, adding more ghee as needed.

7. **To make the aioli**, mix the mayonnaise with the minced garlic and serve on the side or on top of the fish cakes.

Cheesy Baked Sea Scallops

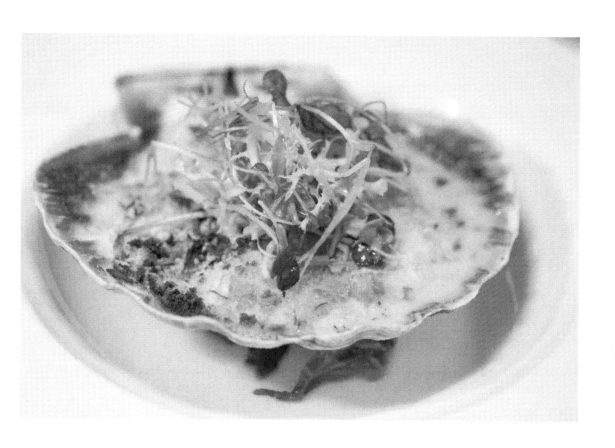

Nutritional Information Per Serving			
Yield:	10 servings	Serving Size:	1 scallop
Calories:	170	Fat:	13 grams
Carbohydrates:	3 grams	Protein:	11 grams
Fiber	0 grams		

Cheesy Baked Sea Scallops

If you're hesitant to try cooking scallops, this recipe is just what you need. Scallops are not hard to do right; they just take a little attention. This recipe combines cheese to with pork rinds and jalapenos for a bright pop of flavor. Despite the recipe's recommended serving size, it wouldn't be too outrageous to serve two or three scallops to each person.

Ingredients:

- 10 sea scallops, in their shells

- 1 lemon, juiced

- 2 tablespoons water

- 2 tablespoons butter

- 4 cloves garlic, peeled and chopped fine

- ⅓ cup grated cheddar cheese

- ¾ cup shredded Mozzarella

- ⅓ cup pork rinds

- ⅓ cup heavy cream

- 2 jalapeno peppers, seeded and sliced thin

- 2 lemons, juiced

Directions:

1. Preheat oven to 400 degrees Fahrenheit.

2. Remove the scallops from their shells.

3. Combine the juice of a lemon with the water and brush on the scallops. This will get rid of any fishy smell.

4. Fill a bowl with hot water and drop the scallops in, soaking them for 15 minutes.

5. Prepare a baking tray with foil.

6. Wipe the scallop shells with a clean kitchen towel and place them on the baking sheet.

7. Take the scallops from the water and dab them dry with a paper towel. Then set each one in a shell. Sprinkle lightly with salt.

8. Bake for five minutes and drain the broth from the tray.

9. In a skillet, over low heat, melt the butter and sauté the garlic until golden.

10. Combine the cheddar and Mozzarella cheeses in a bowl. Crush the pork rinds and add to the cheese.

11. Pour ½ teaspoon of butter over each scallop in its shell. Sprinkle with the cheese and pork rind mixture and top with a slice of jalapeno.

12. Bake for eight to 10 minutes or until the cheese is melted.

Clam Chowder À La Crock-Pot

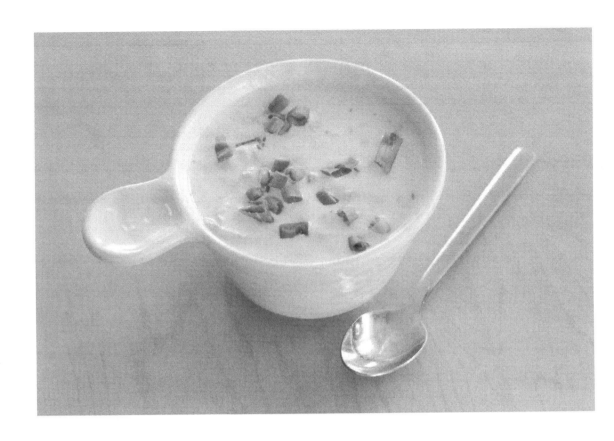

Nutritional Information Per Serving			
Yield:	12 servings	Serving Size:	¼ ounce
Calories:	276	Fat:	29 grams
Carbohydrates:	13 grams	Protein:	12 grams
Fiber	1 gram		

Ketogenic Clam Chowder

You will want to eat all 12 servings yourself because this chowder is absolutely delicious. It does include the smoky flavor of bacon, but you can leave that out if you want. Not much has to be done with this recipe except dump everything in the Crock-Pot and let it go. You do have to put some of the ingredients on and then wait an hour before adding the rest, but if you get up early in the morning, you can put it on, get dressed and ready, and add the rest of the ingredients before heading out the door.

Ingredients:

- ¼ cup chicken stock

- 3 green onions, thinly sliced

- 3 cloves garlic, peeled and minced

- 2 ribs celery, thinly sliced

- 1 medium yellow onion, peeled and chopped

- 2 tablespoons butter

- 1 teaspoon black pepper

- ½ teaspoon sea salt

- 3 10-ounce cans fancy whole baby clams, drained (save juice)

- 2 cups clam juice (add water to the above juice to make two cups)

- 1-pound thick-cut bacon, cooked and crumbled

- 1½ cups heavy cream

- 1 8-ounce brick cream cheese, softened

- ½ teaspoon dry thyme

- ½ teaspoon garlic powder

Directions:

1. Put the chicken stock, garlic, green onion, celery, yellow onion, butter, salt, and pepper into a slow cooker. Cover and cook on the low setting for one hour.

2. Add the clams, clam juice, bacon, cream, cream cheese, thyme, and garlic powder. Mix until the smooth with no lumps of cream cheese.

3. Cover and cook on low for six to eight hours. Serve hot.

Fuss-Free Foil-Baked Halibut

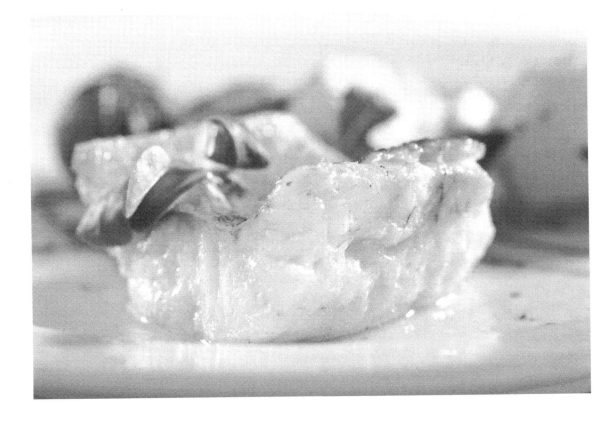

Nutritional Information Per Serving			
Yield:	2 servings	Serving Size:	½ fillet
Calories:	119	Fat:	3 grams
Carbohydrates:	0 grams	Protein:	23 grams
Fiber	0 grams		

Baked Halibut

This dish is fuss-free because you combine all the ingredients in foil, fold it up, put it on the grill to cook, then eat it. There are hardly any dishes to wash unless you make a side dish. This recipe celebrates the unadulterated flavor of the halibut.

Ingredients:

- 1 6-ounce halibut fillet

- salt and pepper to taste

- ½ teaspoon garlic powder

- ½ teaspoon onion powder

- any other herb or spice you might like to include

Directions:

1. Lay a piece of foil flat with the shiny side on the counter and cover with non-stick spray.

2. Season the fillet with herbs and spices.

3. Wrap the two long ends together, fold in the sides, and seal all seams so the fish is airtight.

4. Place the foil package on the grill over medium heat.

5. Grill for eight minutes. When the halibut is white and flakes, it is done.

Keto Fish Nuggets

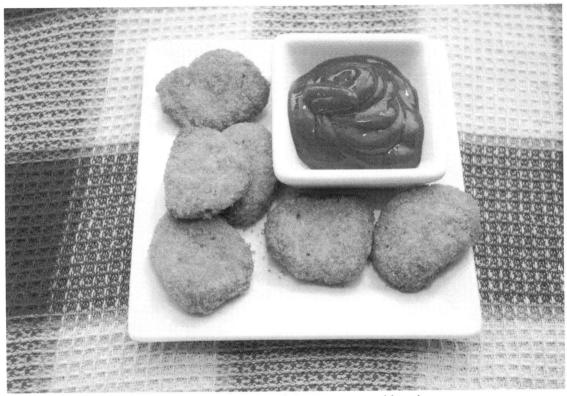

Fish nuggets, served with keto-approved ketchup

Nutritional Information Per Serving			
Yield:	3 servings	Serving Size:	10 nuggets
Calories:	433	Fat:	24 grams
Carbohydrates:	0 grams	Protein:	51 grams
Fiber	0 grams		

Keto Fish Nuggets

Kids and adults alike just love these nuggets. The "breading" uses pork rinds and Parmesan cheese; you'll find it simply delicious. The recipe calls for frozen tilapia fillets, but I do not particularly like tilapia. I use any firm fish fillet like catfish or flounder. I have even used halibut and found it held up pretty well.

Ingredients:

- 3 tilapia fillets, thawed

- ½ cup pork rinds

- ½ cup Parmesan cheese

- ¼ teaspoon cayenne pepper

- 1 teaspoon garlic powder

- ½ teaspoon salt

- ¼ teaspoon pepper

- 1 egg

- 1 tablespoon heavy cream

- Olive oil

Directions:

1. Place the pork rinds in a food processor or blender and grind into a fine powder.

2. Mix the pork rind powder and Parmesan cheese in a bowl along with the cayenne pepper, garlic powder, salt, and pepper.

3. In another bowl, whisk together the egg and heavy cream.

4. Cut the fish into 1-inch squares. Do not cut them smaller or they will too easily overcook.

5. Heat a skillet and add olive oil, covering the bottom by a quarter inch.

6. Coat each fish piece in the egg mixture and roll it in the pork rind mixture.

7. Place it in the oil and fry until golden brown, which will take two to three minutes, flipping the nugget halfway through.

Keto Shrimp Scampi

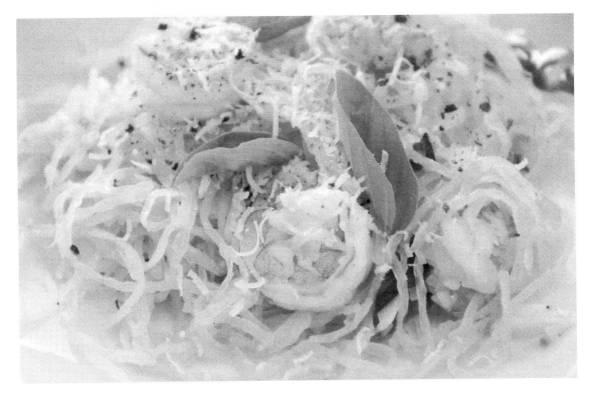

Nutritional Information Per Serving			
Yield:	2 servings	Serving Size:	2 cups
Calories:	276	Fat:	11 grams
Carbohydrates:	6 grams	Protein:	31 grams
Fiber	1.7 grams		

Keto Shrimp Scampi

This little shrimp recipe is delicious. Better yet, it requires only a few minutes of stovetop cooking. It pairs well with the spaghetti squash.

Here is a helpful hint: This recipe uses both olive o[i]
The olive oil prevents the butter from getting brown t
works with recipes that require a hot skillet. You will
butter if you add olive oil, too.

Ingredients:

- 2 tablespoons olive oil

- 2 tablespoons butter

- 1 tablespoon minced garlic

- ½ cup dry white wine

- ¼ teaspoon red pepper flakes

- ½ teaspoon salt (kosher or sea salt)

- ⅛ teaspoon ground black pepper

- 2 pounds shrimp, deveined and peeled

- 2 tablespoons lemon juice

- 1 teaspoon lemon zest

- ⅓ cup fresh parsley, chopped

- 3 cups spaghetti squash, cooked

Directions:

1. Heat a sauté pan on the stove and add the olive oil and butter.

2. Cook the garlic in the pan for about two to three minutes. The butter and olive oil combination will prevent it from turning too brown.

3. Add the wine, red pepper flakes, salt and pepper and cook two minutes stirring.

4. Add the shrimp and cook two to three minutes, stirring until they turn opaque.

5. Remove from the heat and add the lemon juice, lemon zest, and parsley.

6. Serve atop a bed of spaghetti squash.

Low-Carb – Yes, It Is Possible – Lobster Roll

Nutritional Information Per Serving			
Yield:	2 servings	Serving Size:	1 roll
Calories:	100	Fat:	4 grams
Carbohydrates:	5 grams	Protein:	13 grams
Fiber	1 gram		

I love lobster rolls and feared my days of enjoying them had come to an end, until I discovered this recipe. Instead of bread, you use a leaf of lettuce, which I find more tasty, crunchy, and flavorful. Place your lettuce leaves in a bowl of cold water about 15 minutes before you start, and then remove them and set on paper towels to dry while you make the lobster mixture. They will stay nice and crisp, giving you a nice crunch when you bite down.

Ingredients:

*   2 tablespoons mayonnaise (see recipe in the next chapter)

*   12 ounces lobster meat, cooked

*   1 cup celery, chopped fine

*   1 teaspoon fresh chopped tarragon

*   1 teaspoon fresh chopped chives

- 1 teaspoon fresh squeezed lemon juice

- 2 romaine lettuce leaves

- Salt and pepper to taste

Directions:

1. Place the mayonnaise in a bowl and add the cooked lobster meat. Stir to combine.

2. Add the celery, tarragon, chives, and lemon juice and combine well.

3. Flatten out a lettuce leaf and spoon the lobster mixture onto the curve of the leaf.

4. Fold and serve.

Pan-Seared Butter Salmon

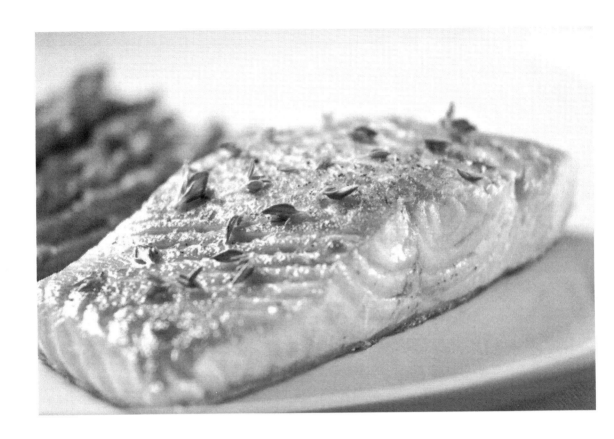

Nutritional Information Per Serving			
Yield:	2 servings	Serving Size:	1 fillet
Calories:	435	Fat:	31 grams
Carbohydrates:	5 grams	Protein:	29 grams
Fiber	2 grams		

Pan-Seared Butter Salmon

This dish has a variety of flavors that I like together. Salmon is a strong flavor in itself, but this dish involves mushrooms and also a buttery, balsamic tomato sauce with lots of garlic and spinach. It pairs well with the salmon and makes a feast. The best thing about this recipe is that it takes less than 30 minutes to prepare and place on the table.

Ingredients:

- 2 salmon fillets

- salt and pepper to taste

- 2 tablespoons olive oil, divided

- 2 cloves garlic, peeled and minced

- ½ pound mushrooms, cleaned and sliced

- 2-3 roma tomatoes, chopped

- 2 tablespoons butter

- 2 cups fresh spinach

- 1 teaspoon balsamic vinegar

Directions:

1. Pat the salmon fillets with a paper towel to dry them off. Season each side with salt and pepper and put them on a plate in the refrigerator while preparing the rest of the recipe.

2. Place a skillet over medium heat and add one tablespoon of the olive oil. Once it is heated, add garlic and mushrooms and cook for three to four minutes.

3. Add butter and let it melt.

4. Add the tomatoes and cook them down a bit.

5. Add the spinach and let it wilt.

6. Place the veggies in a bowl, cover with foil to keep warm and set aside.

7. In the same skillet, add the other tablespoon of olive oil and get it very hot.

8. Remove the salmon from the refrigerator and set it in the pan, skin-side down, and sear for four to five minutes. Do not turn or disturb.

9. Flip and sear for another four to five minutes.

10. Uncover the vegetables and drizzle with balsamic vinegar.

11. Put some on a plate and top with the salmon. You can use a little lemon juice on top and garnish with a lemon slice if you desire.

Super Simple Crab Vegetable Omelet Casserole

Nutritional Information Per Serving			
Yield:	15 servings	Serving Size:	147 grams
Calories:	141	Fat:	8 grams
Carbohydrates:	4 grams	Protein:	14 grams
Fiber	2 grams		

This recipe is more like a big vegetable and crab omelet, but it is delicious. I like using fresh crab that has been cooked, but you can also use canned or frozen crab to make things go faster. The best thing about this recipe is that you can swap out any of the vegetables you don't like for ones you do.

Ingredients:

- 8 large eggs

- 2 cups almond milk

- 1 small eggplant, chopped

- 1 green pepper, seeded and chopped

- 1 red pepper, seeded and chopped

- 1 small onion, peeled and chopped or three green onions, chopped

- 1-pound crabmeat, chopped

- 4 ounces Swiss cheese, shredded or chopped

- 1 cup cheddar cheese, shredded

- ½ teaspoon black pepper, ground

- 1 teaspoon Old Bay seasoning

Directions:

1. Preheat the oven to 350 degrees Fahrenheit and coat a 13 by 9-inch baking pan with non-stick spray.

2. Beat the eggs in a large bowl and add the almond milk, beating well.

3. Prepare all the vegetables and put them in the bowl with the egg mixture and the crabmeat.

4. Add the cheeses to the bowl and mix well.

5. Add the pepper and Old Bay seasoning and incorporate well.

6. Pour the mixture into the baking dish and bake for 40 to 45 minutes or until a knife inserted in the center comes out clean.

7. Do not cut until at least 10 to 15 minutes have passed. If you do, the casserole will be flat instead of fluffy and light.

Many of the recipes in this book call for other dished to make an entire meal, such as zucchini noodles or cauliflower rice. The next chapter details these side dishes and other accents needed to finish out a meal.

Chapter 10: Sides and Sauces

Some of the main dish recipes in this book mention other foods that are used as accompaniments or side dishes. Mayonnaise or ketchup often accompany other dishes or are used as an ingredient in a recipe. Since noodles and rice are taboo in this diet, it helps to have alternatives that you can eat, either as side dishes or as foundations for other items that traditionally call for them. That's what this chapter is all about.

Here, you will learn how to make potato salad, mushroom pilaf, and macaroni and cheese, using cauliflower. You'll make fries from green beans and zucchini. You will also learn how to make a loaf of bread, hamburger buns, and tortillas, using low-carb ingredients. If you love gravy, do not despair; you'll find several delicious recipes that will tantalize your taste buds while meeting your macros.

Aioli

Nutritional Information Per Serving			
Yield:	25 servings	Serving Size:	1 Tablespoon
Calories:	145	Fat:	17 grams
Carbohydrates:	0.3 grams	Protein:	0.3 grams
Fiber	0.03 grams		

This versatile sauce is at times part mayonnaise, part tartar sauce, or part dip, and at all times delicious. Try it on fish, poultry, on Italian dishes. Add a dollop atop soups, serve aside pork. You can experiment with it virtually anywhere, with positive results.

Ingredients:

- 5 cloves garlic

- 1 egg

220

- 1 tablespoon Dijon mustard

- 1¾ cup olive oil

- Salt to taste

- Pepper to taste

- Lemon juice, fresh, as needed to adjust the sauce thickness per preference

Directions:

1. Dip the garlic cloves in the olive oil, place on a small baking dish, and roast in a 400-degree Fahrenheit oven for about 10 minutes, until soft and slightly browned.

2. Set the garlic aside to cool.

3. Combine in a blender, the egg, mustard, salt, and pepper; add the cooled garlic and blend thoroughly until smooth.

4. Gradually add in the olive oil while blending, until completely combined.

5. If you prefer a thinner texture, add lemon juice until the sauce reaches your preferred consistency.

6. Store in an airtight container in the refrigerator. The mixture should be good for about three weeks.

Faux Macaroni And Cheese

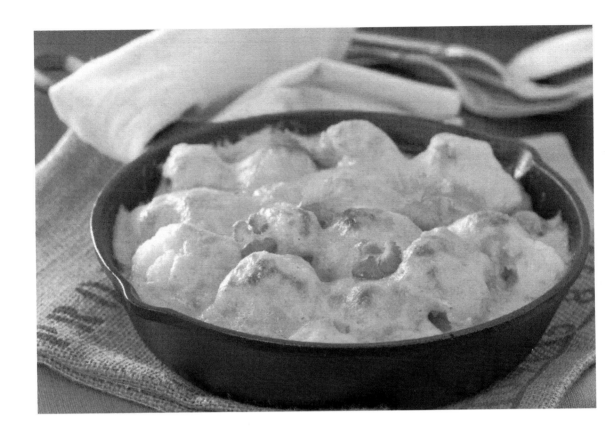

Nutritional Information Per Serving			
Yield:	8 servings	Serving Size:	¾ cup
Calories:	296	Fat:	25 grams
Carbohydrates:	5 grams	Protein:	11 grams
Fiber	2.6 grams		

Faux Macaroni and Cheese 1

Some dishes are hard to give up, especially when you grow up with them. Macaroni and cheese is one of those for me. This "macaroni" is made from cauliflower. Although it doesn't taste *exactly* like the old pasta-laden standby, the dish is close enough to stand on its own merits.

Ingredients:

- 2 pounds frozen cauliflower florets

- 1 cup heavy whipping cream

- 1 4-ounce brick of cream cheese, cubed

- 8 ounces shredded cheddar cheese, divided

- 1 teaspoon turmeric

- ½ teaspoon garlic powder

- 1 teaspoon Dijon mustard

- Salt and pepper to taste

Directions:

1. Cook the cauliflower in boiling water as per package instructions. Drain well.

2. In a large pan over medium heat, bring the cream to a simmer. Once it starts to bubble, add the cream cheese and stir with a wire whisk until it becomes smooth.

3. Add six ounces of the shredded cheddar cheese and mix in well. Save the other two ounces for later.

4. Add the turmeric, garlic powder, Dijon mustard, salt, and pepper. The sauce will smooth out and turn a light yellow color.

5. Add the drained cauliflower to the cheese sauce and make sure all florets are coated.

6. Sprinkle with the rest of the shredded cheese and wait until mostly melted before stirring.

7. Serve hot.

Faux Mashed Potatoes

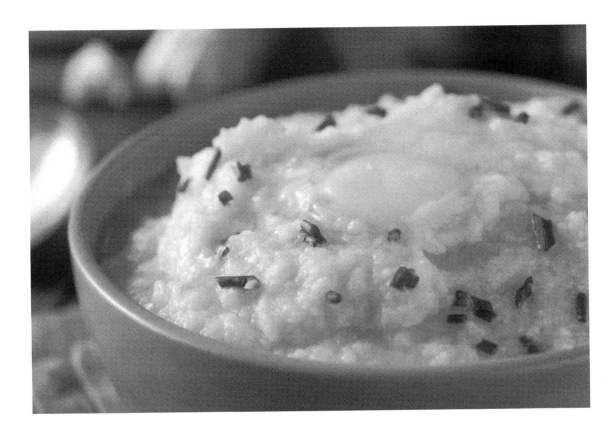

Nutritional Information Per Serving			
Yield:	6 servings	Serving Size:	~1 cup
Calories:	244	Fat:	23 grams
Carbohydrates:	5 grams	Protein:	6 grams
Fiber	3 grams		

Faux Mashed Potatoes

I really miss mashed potatoes, so I make something out of cauliflower that looks like it; it even has a similar texture. The end result tastes a little different, but is delicious, nonetheless. It only takes about 10 minutes to make up and this recipe turns out creamy and delicious.

Ingredients:

- 20 ounces of riced cauliflower (see cauliflower rice recipe, this chapter)

- ½ cup sour cream

- ¼ cup heavy whipping cream

- 6 tablespoons butter

- ½ cup grated Parmesan cheese

- ½ teaspoon garlic powder

- salt and pepper to taste

Directions:

1. Place riced cauliflower in a microwave safe bowl and cover with a paper towel. Microwave on high for five minutes.

2. The rice should be somewhat firm but soft to the touch.

3. Mix in the sour cream, whipping cream, butter, Parmesan, garlic powder and salt and pepper.

4. It will be lumpy. Use an immersion blender to make it creamy and smooth.

5. Top with gravy.

Faux Rice, a.k.a., Riced Cauliflower

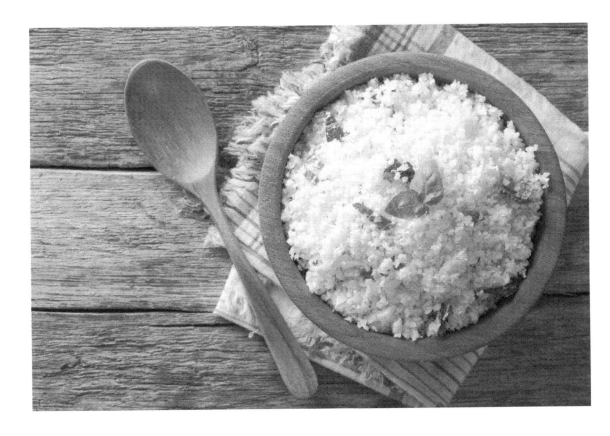

Nutritional Information Per Serving			
Yield:	varies	Serving Size:	1 cup
Calories:	25	Fat:	0.3 grams
Carbohydrates:	5 grams	Protein:	1.9 grams
Fiber	2 grams		

Faux rice, made from cauliflower

White and brown rice are full of carbs, so when you have a recipe that calls for rice, this recipe offers a low-carb alternative. Here is how to make it:

1. Clean a head of cauliflower by removing the leaves.

2. Cut the head into florets and place them in a colander. Rinse well and let drain well.

3. Wait until the cauliflower dries to proceed or you will have a soggy mess to deal with.

4. Use the grating blade in your food processor and pulse after each addition of florets so you end up with something that looks like rice.

5. Put the "rice" in an air tight bowl and store in the refrigerator until you are ready to use it.

How to use cauliflower rice:

1. Steam the cauliflower rice in a steam pot for five to seven minutes.

2. Place the rice in a microwave safe bowl and cook on medium for five to seven minutes. Do not add any water.

3. Put a tablespoon of butter or ghee in a saucepan and warm it up.

4. Preheat your oven to 400 degrees Fahrenheit. Cover a baking sheet with parchment paper and spread the rice over it. Use a baking sheet with sides or the rice will spread everywhere. After eight minutes stir it around and put it back in for another eight minutes.

Faux Tater Tots

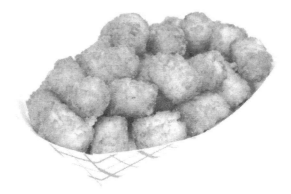

Nutritional Information Per Serving			
Yield:	4 servings	Serving Size:	9 tots
Calories:	236	Fat:	18 grams
Carbohydrates:	6 grams	Protein:	9 grams
Fiber	0 grams		

Faux Tater Tots

Tater tots were always a favorite when I was growing up; they still are. You can imagine how glad I was to learn I could make them out of cauliflower with just a fraction of the carbs and much more flavor.

Ingredients:

- 1 medium head of cauliflower

- 2 ounces shredded Mozzarella cheese

- ¼ cup grated Parmesan cheese

- 1 large egg

- 2 teaspoons psyllium husk powder

- ½ teaspoon onion powder

- ½ teaspoon garlic powder

- Salt and pepper to taste

- 1 cup oil or bacon fat

Directions:

1. Cut the cauliflower into florets and discard any long fibrous stems.

2. Steam the florets until they are tender. Put florets in a food processor and pulse until the consistency of mashed potatoes.

3. Place the cauliflower in a clean dish towel and squeeze out as much moisture as you can. Place in a bowl and let it cool.

4. Add the Parmesan cheese, Mozzarella cheese, and the egg to the bowl and mix well with a spoon. Add the psyllium husk powder, onion, and garlic powder and season to taste with salt and pepper. Mix everything thoroughly.

5. Take a teaspoon of the mixture and form it into a ball with your hand, then shape it into a log. Press the two ends together to make a tot shape. Do this with all of the mixture.

6. Heat the oil or bacon fat in a cast iron skillet over medium heat. Reduce to low heat and add the tater tots, about six at a time. Turn so they become crisp on all sides.

7. Drain briefly on paper towels and serve.

Fried Green Beans

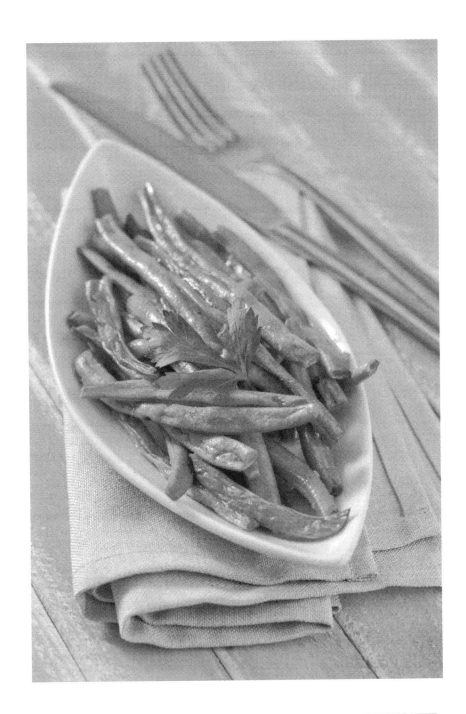

Nutritional Information Per Serving			
Yield:	4 servings	Serving Size:	1 cup
Calories:	113	Fat:	7 grams

Carbohydrates:	11 grams	Protein:	3 grams
Fiber	1.4 grams		

Fried Green Beans

Fried green beans make a delicious substitute for French fries. The beans come out crispy and covered with a delicious garlicky Parmesan cheese coating. You do need to make them with whole fresh green beans; canned or frozen just won't do in this case.

Ingredients:

- 12 ounces fresh green beans

- ⅔ cup Parmesan cheese, grated

- ½ teaspoon garlic powder

- ¼ teaspoon paprika

- ½ teaspoon sea salt

- ¼ teaspoon black pepper, ground

- 1 large egg, beaten

Directions:

1. Preheat the oven to 400 degrees Fahrenheit.

2. Prepare a large baking sheet by lining it with parchment paper, and coating with non-stick spray.

3. Prepare green beans by trimming the ends and washing them. Make sure they are completely dry before going any further.

4. In a shallow bowl, combine the Parmesan cheese, garlic powder, paprika, sea salt, and pepper and mix well.

5. In a large bowl, whisk the egg until frothy.

6. Grab a handful of the beans and drop them into the bowl with the egg. Stir with your hands to thoroughly coat, then take the bunch out by hand, letting them drip for a few seconds. Give them a shake and put them in the shallow bowl with the Parmesan mixture.

7. Press the coated beans in to the Parmesan mixture to coat well on all sides.

8. Place the beans on the baking sheet, making sure they do not overlap. You might need to use two baking sheets. Continue with the rest of the beans. If you start running out of egg, just use another one.

9. Put them in the preheated oven and bake for 10 minutes or until the cheese is slightly golden.

10. Remove from the oven and cool for 10 minutes on the baking sheet.

11. Serve as is or with a Ranch dressing dipping sauce.

Hot Asian Broccoli Salad

Nutritional Information Per Serving			
Yield:	8 servings	Serving Size:	~1 cup
Calories:	62	Fat:	4 grams
Carbohydrates:	4.7 grams	Protein:	2 grams
Fiber	1.1 grams		

This is a nice option for a low-carb side dish that is hearty and warm. It is low in carbohydrates, but high in flavor. You'll enjoy the contrast between the smooth and creamy, the gingery tang, and the crunch of sesame seeds.

Ingredients:

- 2 tablespoons coconut oil

- 1 12-ounce bag broccoli slaw

- 1 tablespoon coconut aminos

- ¼ teaspoon salt

- ¼ teaspoon pepper

- 1 teaspoon fresh ginger, grated from a finger of ginger

- ½ cup full fat plain goat milk yogurt (cow milk yogurt doesn't taste the same)

- ½ tablespoon sesame seeds

Directions:

1. Place a skillet over medium high heat and add the coconut oil. Pour the broccoli slaw in, cover the skillet and cook for seven minutes.

2. Uncover and stir in the aminos, salt, pepper, and ginger.

3. Remove from heat and add the yogurt and sesame seeds, stirring them in well.

4. Serve warm as a side dish.

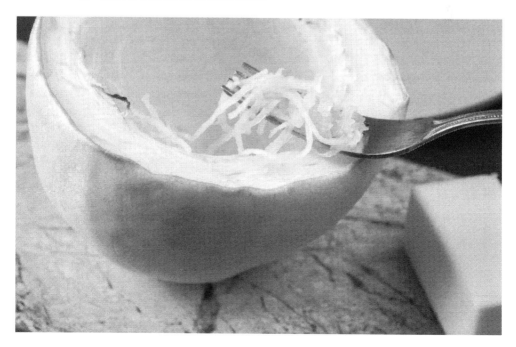

How To Cook Spaghetti Squash

Nutritional Information Per Serving			
Yield:	varies	Serving Size:	1 cup
Calories:	31	Fat:	0.6 grams
Carbohydrates:	7 grams	Protein:	0.6 grams
Fiber	1.5 grams		

Spaghetti Squash

Of course, pasta is a big no-no in low-carb diets and many of the recipes in this book use spaghetti squash instead. Spaghetti squash is an oblong yellow–orange squash that, when cooked, produces strands that resemble pasta. It is super easy to prepare and use in recipes.

Ingredients:

- Spaghetti squash

- Olive oil

- Sea salt

Directions:

1. Preheat the oven to 400 degrees Fahrenheit.

2. Cut the squash in half, then scoop out and discard the seeds.

3. Drizzle each half with a liberal amount of olive oil and sprinkle with salt.

4. Place a piece of parchment paper on a baking sheet and place the squash, cut side down on the baking sheet.

5. Roast for 45 to 50 minutes.

6. Remove from the oven and let cool about 10 minutes.

7. Turn the squash over and use a fork to scrape out the strands.

Keto Buns

Nutritional Information Per Serving			
Yield:	1 serving	Serving Size:	1 bun
Calories:	248	Fat:	20 grams
Carbohydrates:	10.7grams	Protein:	8 grams
Fiber	7.7 grams		

I crave a good old hamburger occasionally and just eating a patty doesn't do it. I want that tactile sensation of eating the hamburger with my hands wrapped around a bun. This recipe only makes one bun, so you will want to increase it, based on how many buns you want. Make each bun separately. Don't make any that will be left over because they don't stay fresh very long. The bun does not taste exactly like a hamburger bun, but when you put the patty inside, it will satisfy that craving for a hamburger.

You will need a wide mouth mug for this one and you will cook it in the microwave. The recipe calls for psyllium husk powder, readily available in health food stores.

Ingredients:

- 1 large egg

- 1 tablespoon melted butter

- 1 tablespoon almond flour

- 1 tablespoon psyllium husk powder

- ¼ teaspoon cream of tartar

- 1 tablespoon chicken broth

Directions:

1. Crack the egg into a large-mouthed mug.

2. Pour the hot melted butter over top of the egg and use a fork to mix well.

3. Add the rest of the ingredients and mix well. The batter will be doughy. Smooth the top down so it is flat in the bottom of the mug and wipe any excess dough from the sides of the mug.

4. Microwave 60 to 75 seconds. The dough will puff up quickly but will fall when you remove it from the microwave.

5. Remove from microwave and turn upside down tapping the opening lightly against a plate. The bun should fall out.

6. Cut bun in half, swirl a little butter in a sauté pan and sauté until it browns.

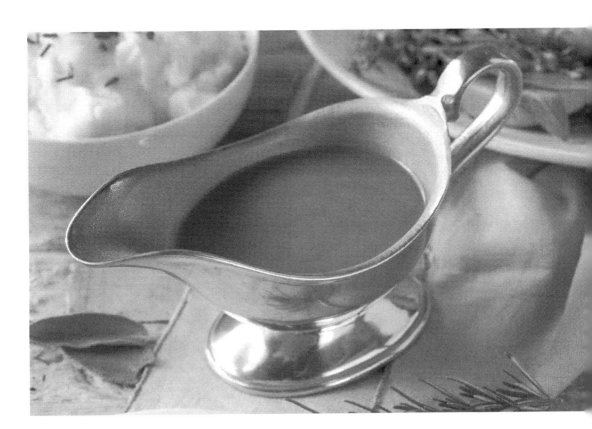

Keto Gravy

Keto Gravy

I suppose you gave up your dreams of rich gravy when you had to let go of your precious mashed potatoes. Fortunately, we can easily get around the high-carb thickeners by using items like cream, sour cream, coconut flour, and vegetable gums, these last available at your health food store.

This recipe works well as a delicious low-carb version of gravy. I use chicken or turkey stock when making poultry gravy and beef broth when making gravy for roasts and other beef dishes.

Ingredients:

- Pan drippings from cooked meat

- 1 stick butter (or ½ cup coconut oil)

- 1 clove garlic, peeled and minced

- 2 cups broth

- 1 tablespoon coconut flour

- ¼ cup heavy whipping cream

- 1 teaspoon Dijon mustard (omit with poultry)

- 2 sprigs fresh thyme

- ¼ teaspoon sea salt

- 1 dash fresh ground pepper

Directions:

1. Strain the pan drippings and set aside.

2. Drop the butter in a large saucepan and melt over low heat.

3. Drop in the garlic and fry for a minute.

4. Add the pan drippings and stir to combine.

5. Add the broth and blend with a whisk over medium high heat.

6. Whisk in the coconut flour and simmer for five to 10 minutes.

7. Remove from heat and whisk in the cream, Dijon mustard, thyme, salt, and pepper.

8. Use an immersion blender to get a smooth consistency and serve with your main dish.

Keto-Approved Ketchup

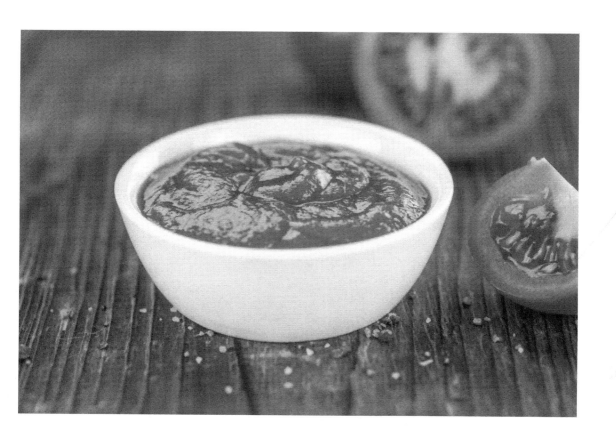

Nutritional Information Per Serving			
Yield:	32 servings	Serving Size:	1 tablespoon
Calories:	5	Fat:	1 gram
Carbohydrates:	1 gram	Protein:	1 gram
Fiber	0.2 grams		

Ketogenic Ketchup

On tablespoon is considered a serving of this delicious ketchup and the recipe makes two cups. I put this in a canning jar, and it keeps in the refrigerator for about one month.

Ingredients:

- 2 cloves garlic, peeled and minced

- 1 small onion, peeled and chopped

- 1 cup tomato puree

- ¼ cup apple cider vinegar

- ⅛ teaspoon allspice

- ⅛ teaspoon ground cloves

- 4 drops stevia

- 2 tablespoons Swerve

- 1 teaspoon sea salt

- 1 pinch ground pepper

- ¼ cup water (approximately; vary to adjust the thickness to your liking)

Directions:

1. Peel and chop the garlic and onion and place in a saucepan along with the rest of the ingredients, except the water, and bring to a boil.

2. Reduce the heat to low and simmer for 10 minutes, adding water if it becomes too thick.

3. Place the contents of the pan in a blender or use an immersion blender to process until smooth.

4. Pour into a jar and let it cool before covering and storing in the refrigerator.

Keto-Approved Sausage Gravy (Country Gravy)

Nutritional Information Per Serving			
Yield:	4 servings	Serving Size:	1 cup
Calories:	277	Fat:	36 grams
Carbohydrates:	2.2 grams	Protein:	5.8 grams

Fiber	0.4 grams	

My family loves country gravy made with sausage and they usually serve it over biscuits, but we now use it over chicken fried steak and mashed cauliflower. This recipe uses guar gum and heavy cream to do the thickening.

Ingredients:

- 4 ounces country sausage

- 2 tablespoons butter

- 1 cup heavy cream

- ½ teaspoon guar gum

- salt and pepper

Directions:

1. Brown the sausage well all the way through in a large skillet and use a slotted spoon to remove the sausage to a bowl when done.

2. Add the butter to the pan and allow it to melt.

3. Add the cream to the pan and stir. Let it come to a bubble.

4. Add the guar gum and stir with a whisk vigorously while it continues to bubble. The mixture should thicken to the point where you run a spatula through the gravy and it takes a while for the gap to close on the bottom of the pan.

5. Put the sausage back in the pan and stir.

Ketogenic Bread

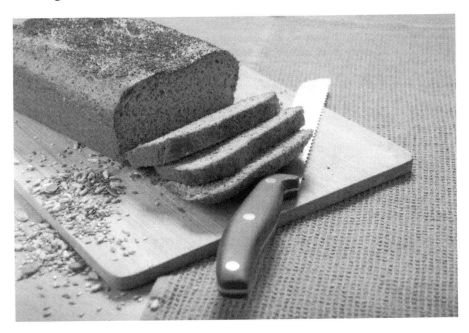

Nutritional Information Per Serving			
Yield:	8 servings	Serving Size:	1 slice
Calories:	134	Fat:	8 grams
Carbohydrates:	3 grams	Protein:	8 grams
Fiber	1.5 grams		

Ketogenic Bread

I use a regular loaf pan to make this bread and it cuts nicely into slices. It has a nutty flavor that is very pleasant, and the batter is much less sticky than bread made with flour. It is very thick and dense, but it bakes up very light.

Ingredients:

- 1 cup coconut flour, sifted

- 1 teaspoon salt

- 1 teaspoon baking powder

- ½ teaspoon baking soda

- ½ cup flaxseed meal

- 6 large eggs, room temperature

- 1 tablespoon apple cider vinegar

- ½ cup room temp tap water

Directions:

1. Preheat oven to 350 degrees and grease a standard size loaf pan or two mini loaf pans.

2. Sift the coconut flour into a large bowl.

3. Add the salt, baking powder, baking soda, and flaxseed meal and whisk together.

4. In another bowl, combine the eggs, vinegar, and water and whisk well.

5. Add the wet ingredients to the dry gradually, mixing together after each addition. The batter is very thick. You can combine the egg mixture in an electric mixer bowl and add the dry ingredients gradually using a mixer if you wish.

6. Pour the batter into the loaf pan and it press down.

7. Bake for 40 minutes.

8. Completely cool in the pan before removing and slicing.

Ketogenic Mayonnaise

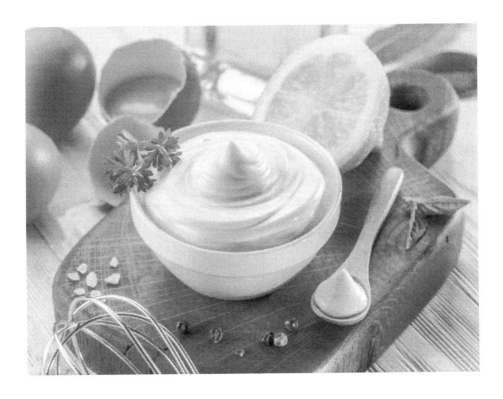

Nutritional Information Per Serving			
Yield:	16 servings	Serving Size:	1 Tbsp.
Calories:	95	Fat:	11 grams
Carbohydrates:	0.2 grams	Protein:	0 grams
Fiber	0 grams		

Ketogenic mayonnaise

You can use this mayonnaise in place of regular mayonnaise or as a dip. This recipe makes one cup of mayo that keeps well for a few weeks in the refrigerator.

Ingredients:

- 1 egg yolk

- ½ lemon, juiced

- 3 tablespoon apple cider vinegar

- ¼ teaspoon paprika

- ¼ teaspoon garlic powder

- ½ teaspoon sea salt

- ¾ cups avocado oil

Directions:

1. Place the egg yolk, lemon juice, vinegar, paprika, garlic powder, and sea salt in a blender and blend for one minute.

2. While still blending, add one tablespoon of the avocado oil into the blender through the opening. Keep adding, one tablespoon at a time so the mixture emulsifies after each addition.

3. Store in an airtight container; this will last for about two weeks.

Low-Carb Tortillas

Nutritional Information Per Serving			
Yield:	10 servings	Serving Size:	1 tortilla
Calories:	132	Fat:	11.8 grams
Carbohydrates:	8 grams	Protein:	2 grams
Fiber	6 grams		

I love taco salad, but there are times you just want to hold a taco in your hand and take a bite out of a tortilla shell. Instead of plain butter, I use half butter and half coconut oil and it seems to hold up a little better than with one or the other. Fill with cheese or taco meat and have a feast.

Ingredients:

- 4 tablespoons psyllium husk powder

- 1 cup coconut flour

- ¼ teaspoon garlic powder

- ½ teaspoon chili powder

- ¼ teaspoon cumin

- ½ cup butter, softened

- 2 cups hot water or chicken broth

Directions:

1. In a large bowl combine the psyllium husk powder, coconut flour, garlic powder, chili powder, and cumin and whisk to combine.

2. Add the softened butter and mix well.

3. Heat the water or broth and add, stirring until everything is melted and well mixed.

4. Shape the dough into a ball and flatten it. Cut into 10 equal wedges.

5. Grease a griddle with coconut oil and heat to medium high. Shape each wedge into a ball.

6. Place a sheet of parchment paper on the counter and flatten the dough ball on it, making it thin. Use another piece of parchment paper on top and a rolling pin if needed.

7. Remove the flattened tortilla from the parchment paper and set it on the griddle to brown the bottom. Flip to the other side and brown. Remove from pan and set aside.

Fill before it cools and hardens. Repeat with the other wedges.

Nutty Roasted Green Beans

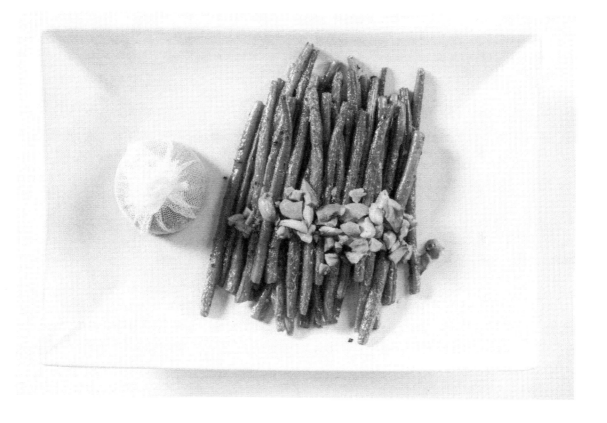

Nutritional Information Per Serving			
Yield:	4 servings	Serving Size:	1 cup
Calories:	336	Fat:	25 grams
Carbohydrates:	11 grams	Protein:	5 grams
Fiber	4.8 grams		

Nutty Roasted Green Beans

I love green beans, especially the ones out of the garden that are crunchy and delicious. This recipe keeps the beans on the crunchy side and the addition of nuts only adds to the crunch. This side is a favorite in my house.

Ingredients:

- 1-pound fresh green beans

- ½ cup chopped pecans, divided

- ¼ cup olive oil

- 2 tablespoons lemon zest

- ¼ cup Parmesan cheese

- 2 teaspoons garlic, peeled and minced

- ½ teaspoon red pepper flakes

Directions:

1. Preheat the oven to 450 degrees.

2. Place the green beans in a large bowl and set aside.

3. Put a quarter cup of pecans into a food processor or blender and grind until they are still a little chunky but mostly mealy.

4. Place the ground pecans, olive oil, lemon zest, Parmesan cheese, minced garlic, and red pepper flakes in the bowl with the green beans and mix them to coat all of the beans.

5. Cover a baking sheet with foil and spread the beans across the baking sheet. They can overlap. Sprinkle the other quarter cup of pecans over the top.

6. Place the beans in the oven for 20 minutes or until roasted. The beans should still be a bit crisp.

7. Let cool for five minutes, then serve while still warm.

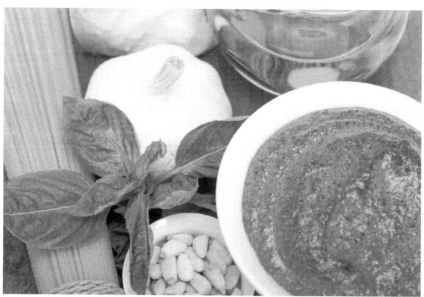

Pesto

Nutritional Information Per Serving			
Yield:	varies	Serving Size:	2 Tablespoons
Calories:	150	Fat:	16 grams
Carbohydrates:	1 gram	Protein:	1 gram
Fiber	1 gram		

Pesto

This fresh pesto will add flavor to any dish. Pesto is a flavorful gift from Italy that can add depth to a wide variety of foods. It doesn't take much to enhance grilled shrimp, steak, or vegetables. A mere dab will enliven even the most staid soups and stews; try it on scrambled eggs and you may never eat your eggs plain again.

The Italian term "pesto" refers to a sauce made of oil, basil, garlic, and cheese. However, there's nothing to say you can't play with these ingredients. The oil is assumed to be olive, but you can substitute avocado oil with no problem. Instead of basil, pesto is frequently made using spinach, parsley, red peppers, or sundried tomatoes. This latter is known as "red pesto."

This recipe doesn't call for cheese, but you can easily add in a quarter cup of grated parmesan cheese to the mix, keeping in mind that the nutritional values will change. The pine nuts in this recipe are purely arbitrary; the dish can be made without (although I like its nutty flavor) or you can substitute any variety of seeds in its place.

Pesto may well become your greatest culinary discovery of the year. Feel free to experiment, both in its use and its contents.

Ingredients:

- 4 cups fresh basil leaves

- ¼ teaspoon sea salt

- ⅛ teaspoon ground pepper

- ½ cup pine nuts

- ½ cup olive oil

- Juice of one lemon

Directions:

1. Place all the ingredients in a food processor.

2. Pulse until creamy, scraping down the sides as needed.

3. If the consistency becomes too thick, feel free to add a little more oil.

Pseudo Wild Rice Mushroom Pilaf

Nutritional Information Per Serving			
Yield:	4 servings	Serving Size:	~1 cup
Calories:	312	Fat:	28 grams
Carbohydrates:	5 grams	Protein:	15 grams
Fiber	2.4 grams		

This recipe will require a trip to the health food store to find shelled hemp heart seeds that you will use as fake rice. Hemp seed is low in carbohydrates and it is slightly crunchier than rice, but I really like the texture. The flavor is different from rice, more earthy, and it complements well the smoky flavor of this dish.

You can use a smoked cheese, such as smoked cheddar or gouda cheese, and omit the liquid smoke, if you prefer.

Ingredients:

- 5 regular-sized mushrooms

- 2 tablespoons butter

- ¼ cup sliced almonds

- 1 cup hemp seeds

- ½ cup chicken broth

- ¼ teaspoon dried parsley

- ½ teaspoon garlic powder

- salt and pepper to taste

Directions:

1. Wash the mushrooms and slice them thinly.

2. Place the butter in a medium sauté pan over medium high heat and let the butter melt.

3. Once it starts to bubble, add the almonds and toast them.

4. Add the mushrooms.

5. When mushrooms are soft, add the hemp seeds and mix together well.

6. Pour in the chicken broth, parsley, garlic powder, salt, and pepper and stir. Turn the heat down to medium low and let everything simmer until the liquid is mostly absorbed.

7. Serve while hot.

Twice-Baked Zucchini

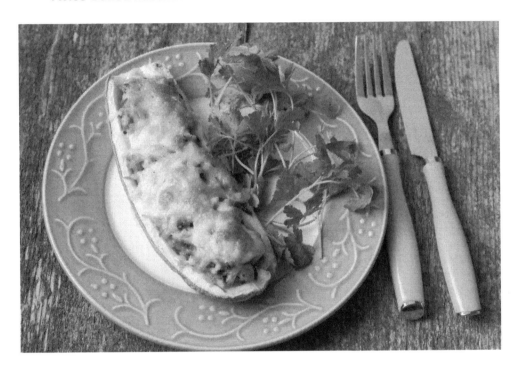

Nutritional Information Per Serving			
Yield:	4 servings	Serving Size:	1 piece
Calories:	260	Fat:	20 grams
Carbohydrates:	7.6 grams	Protein:	7.3 grams
Fiber	1.5 grams		

Twice-baked zucchini

This is a low-carb version of twice baked potatoes, using zucchini. It is just as tasty as the carbohydrate-loaded potato and sometimes I think it tastes even better. It has all the flavor, but it won't weigh you down afterward.

Ingredients:

- 2 medium-sized zucchinis
- 2 tablespoons olive oil
- Salt and pepper to taste
- 4 strips bacon
- ¼ cup yellow or sweet onion, minced
- ½ cup cheddar cheese, shredded
- 2 ounces cream cheese, softened at room temperature
- ¼ cup sour cream
- 2 tablespoons butter, melted
- 1 tablespoon fresh chives, chopped
- Salt and pepper to taste

Directions:

1. Preheat the oven to 350 degrees Fahrenheit.
2. Cut the zucchinis in half lengthwise, opening them up so you can scoop out the seeds.
3. Sprinkle the insides with salt and pepper and drizzle lightly with olive oil. Place the zucchini halves, skin-side up, on a baking sheet and pop into the oven for 15 minutes.
4. Cook the bacon until crisp and set aside to cool.

5. After 15 minutes of baking, pull the pan out of the oven and let the zucchinis cool for five minutes. Then, flip the halves over and gently spoon out the zucchini flesh into a bowl, leaving enough against the skin so that it will hold its shape.

6. Set the skins in a baking dish that has been treated with non-stick spray. Cut up or mash the scooped-out flesh.

7. Add the onion, cheddar cheese, cream cheese, sour cream, and melted butter to the zucchini filling and mix well.

8. Pack the filling into each skin and sprinkle chives and crumbled bacon over the top.

9. Bake for 30 minutes or until the filling starts to bubble. Remove from the oven and cool for 5 minutes before serving.

Zoodles – The Versatile Zucchini Noodle

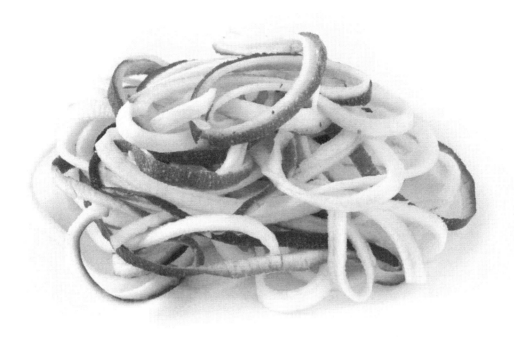

Spiral-cut zucchini

Nutritional Information Per Serving			
Yield:	varies	Serving Size:	1 cup
Calories:	33	Fat:	0.6 grams
Carbohydrates:	6 grams	Protein:	2.4 grams
Fiber	2 grams		

Zucchini Noodles

You can use zucchini noodles, or zoodles, almost anywhere you would normally use noodles. They contain almost no carbs, have only 16 calories per hundred grams, and blend well with any flavor. You may also find them referred to as courgetti, or courgette spaghetti.

There are multiple ways to make zoodles:

- **Use a Spiralizer.** This is a machine that you attach any vegetable to and at the turn of a crank, a blade slices thin spirals. The machine clamps down to your work surface and produces large amounts of spiral-cut veggies in a short time. Children love to turn the crank and watch the amazing spirals magically appear. In addition to the stand-alone spiralizer, you'll find spiralizer attachments to food processors and heavy-duty mixers.

- **Hand-held julienne cutters** look like vegetable peelers but a single swipe down the length of a vegetable will cut a swath of straight strands that will work just as effectively as the spirals; just watch out for the sharp blades, they'll julienne your skin if you aren't careful.

- **Vegetable peeler** – This is how I make my zoodles most of the time, because it is quick and convenient. I can make flat zucchini noodles just by running the vegetable peeler down the length of the zucchini. Some vegetables peelers have a flat side and a julienne side. You can run the julienne side down the zucchini to easily produce noodles. The only problem is that you will have a rather large core when you are done. I usually just cut that up and use it in other recipes.

- **Mandolin** – this is a flat board with a blade. You place the zucchini against the board and run it over the blade to create julienne slices. This works well, but make sure to use the guard to hold the zucchini or you'll find yourself shredding your skin.

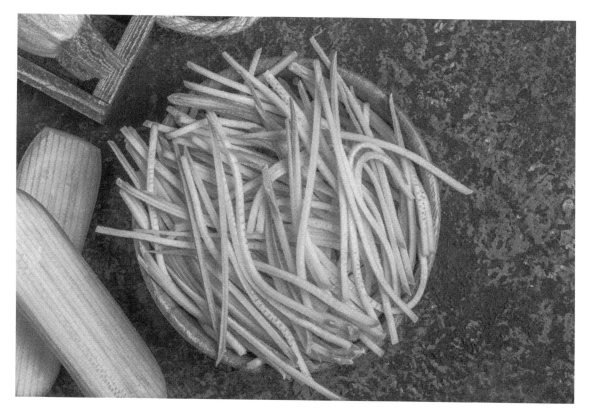

Julienne-cut zucchini

Because the slices you make are very thin and because zucchini is 95% water anyway, they call for special treatment to avoid turning into a limp, soggy mess. Here is how to use your zucchini noodles once you've created them:

- **Use them raw** – I do this often because they are tender just as they are. They add variety and texture to any salad. If I want my dish to be hot, I may plop them in some hot water for a few seconds and drain them just so they are warm. Usually whatever I am serving on top of them is hot enough to warm the noodles, as well.

- **Microwave** – Set the noodles in a microwave-safe dish and heat on high for one minute. This might take a little longer, depending on the number of noodles you are working with. They cook about as quickly as water will come to a boil in the microwave. Then you can doctor them with butter, sour cream, and spices, or eat them plain, however you prefer.

- **Sauté** – Put one tablespoon of olive oil, avocado oil, or butter in a sauté pan to melt, then add the noodles, stirring until they are hot.

- **Boil** – Put a pan of water on and once it boils add the noodles. Let them cook for two minutes, then pour out into a colander to drain. If your noodles come out sticky, they're overcooked. Sorry, but there's not a lot you can do with them. Next time, cook them a little less.

- **Bake** – I hardly ever use this method because it takes so long, but I do like the texture. To use this method, preheat the oven to 200 degrees Fahrenheit and line a baking sheet with paper towels. Spread out the noodles on top and sprinkle them with salt. The salt will draw the liquid out of the zucchini and it will be soaked up by the paper towels. Bake for 10 to 15 minutes and then squeeze out

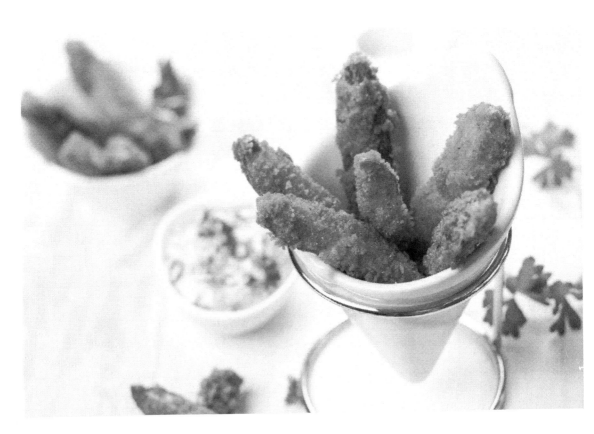

the noodles to get rid of any excess liquid before serving.

Zucchini Parmesan Fries

Nutritional Information Per Serving			
Yield:	4 servings	Serving Size:	8 pieces
Calories:	213	Fat:	15 grams
Carbohydrates:	4 grams	Protein:	21 grams
Fiber	1 gram		

Zucchini Parmesan Fries

These are my favorite fake french fries because they have a texture similar to potato fries. They are made from zucchini, which is readily available, especially in summer. Avoid using really oversized zucchini, because the seeds will get in the way of making this dish. Medium-sized squash, eight or nine inches long work best; I can get 16 sticks out of one.

Ingredients:

- 2 medium sized zucchinis

- 2 large eggs

- ¾ cup grated Parmesan cheese

- ¼ teaspoon sea salt

- ¼ teaspoon ground black pepper

- ¼ teaspoon garlic powder

Directions:

1. Preheat the oven to 425 degrees Fahrenheit and prepare one or two baking sheets by covering them with parchment paper coated with non-stick spray.

2. Cut each zucchini in half lengthwise and again four times to make eight long sticks from each zucchini. Cut all the sticks in half crosswise so your sticks are about four inches long by a half inch thick.

3. Crack the eggs into a bowl and whisk until frothy.

4. In another container, combine the Parmesan cheese, salt, pepper, and garlic powder, mixing well.

5. Dip the zucchini sticks in the egg mixture, then use your hand to scoop them out and shake off the excess egg. Drop them into the dish with the Parmesan mixture and coat all sides of the zucchini sticks.

6. Place the coated sticks on the baking sheet so they do not touch each other.

7. Bake for 15 to 20 minutes, flipping the fries halfway through the baking process. They should appear golden on all sides when finished cooking.

8. Let them cool in the pan for five minutes before serving.

Chapter 11: Easy Meal Plans

It is possible to make any combination of meals out of the recipes in this book. Because each person's nutritional requirements are different, I can't give you a standard meal plan, but I have made up a few to give you a good idea of what you can do.

What A Meal Looks Like

Your ketogenic meals won't look like you're accustomed to. Instead of a main dish, a vegetable, a starch, and maybe a salad for a meal, you'll be eating only one or two items. You won't need to eat a huge amount on this diet, either. Because keto recipes are higher in fat and protein, their calorie count will be higher per portion, and the portion sizes will be smaller than you're probably used to seeing. It's a psychological adjustment, but you'll get used to eating less over time, especially when you aren't getting hungry between meals.

Where To Start

Because you're eating less, it's all the more important that you carefully choose what you eat. Begin with your macros, those all-important numbers that spell out exactly how much you need each day in terms of protein, fat, and carbohydrates. Your body needs those exact amounts of all three. Your challenge will be to balance what you eat so that you include adequate amounts of these nutrients each day.

Unfortunately, since each person needs different levels of protein, fat, and carbohydrates, there's no way I can provide an optimum diet that works for everyone. However, I've given you the nutritional makeup of each of these dishes so you can add the numbers up yourself and turn them into meals that round out your nutritional needs.

Watch Your Ingredients

Keep in mind that these nutritional numbers are approximations that will vary, based on the specific brands you use, and the makeup of the individual components. Meat will vary widely in fat content, and pre-made ingredients will often contain ingredients, especially sugars, that can have a major impact on their carbohydrate content. Over time, you'll become adept and sniffing out ingredients that add hidden carbs to your meals and find ways to avoid them or work around them. That's one reason for creating your own meals from scratch; you know exactly what goes into what you eat and you can adjust the various macronutrients to suit your specific requirements.

Keep track of your macros. You do not want to over-indulge but neither do you want to under-eat. Both extremes can be dangerous. Don't avoid eating because you can't find anything in the house that matches your diet. Plan ahead, make meal plans the week before, and track your macro usage so that you stay healthy and the diet works for you. Many of these dishes freeze well, so you can make extra ahead of time and freeze individual portions for quick reheating later.

That said, here are a few meal ideas that use recipes from this book. Comparing how close the numbers are to yours will give you a starting place for balancing out your day's menu items.

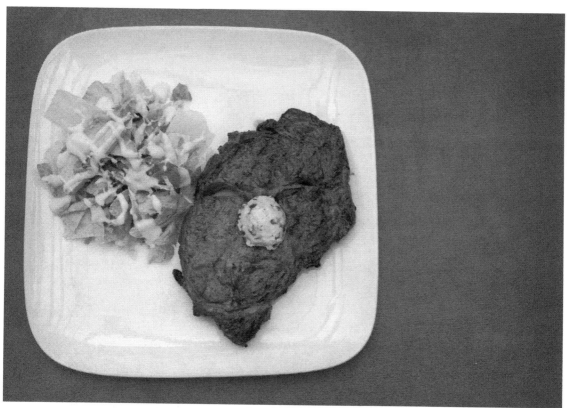

Steak dinner

Beef-Lover's Meal #1

- Cheese-Stuffed Bacon Burger - Chapter 5

- Keto Buns – Chapter 10

- Zucchini Parmesan Fries – Chapter 10

Beef-Lover's Meal #2

- Crock-Pot Beef Pot Roast – Chapter 5

- Green salad with the Zesty Low-Carb Italian Dressing – Chapter 3

263

Beef-Lover's Meal #3

- Ketogenic Steak – Chapter 5

- Cauliflower "Potato" Salad – Chapter 3

- Good-For-You Cream of Broccoli Soup – Chapter 4

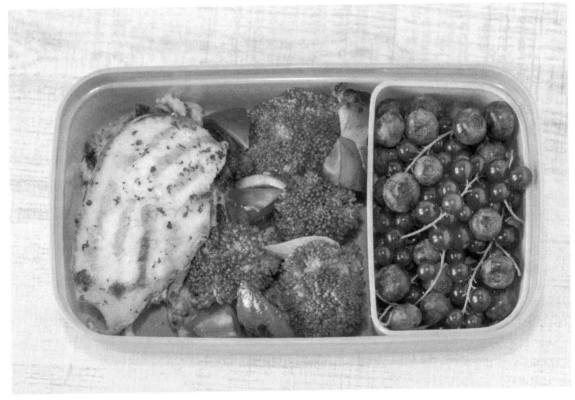

A chicken lunch with fresh vegetables and berries

Poultry-Lover's Meal #1

- Chicken Coconut Curry– Chapter 6

- Pseudo Wild Rice Mushroom Pilaf – Chapter 10

Poultry-Lover's Meal #2

- Simply Smashing Stuffed Chicken Rolls – Chapter 5

- Chicken Zucchini Noodle Soup – Chapter 4

Pork-Lover's Meal #1

- Asian Pork Chops – Chapter 7

- Hot Asian Broccoli Salad – Chapter 10

Pork-Lover's Meal #2

- Bourbon-Glazed Ham – Chapter 7

- Nutty Roasted Green Beans – Chapter 10

- Faux Mashed Potatoes – Chapter 10

Lamb-Lover's Meal #1

- Italian Lamb Chops – Chapter 8

- Pesto – Chapter 10

- Twice Baked Zucchini – Chapter10

Lamb-Lover's Meal #2

- Tender Lamb Shanks À La Crock Pot – Chapter 8

- Fried Green Beans – Chapter 10

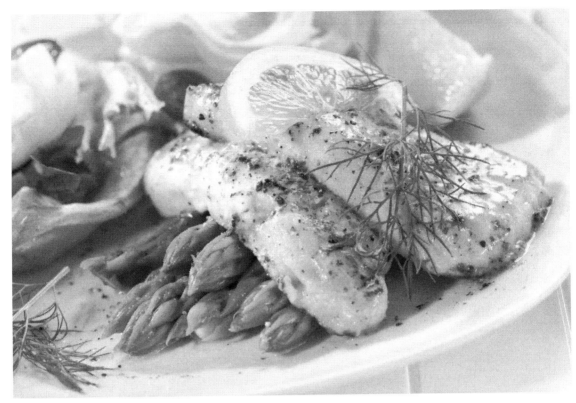

Fish with asparagus

Shrimp-Lover's Meal

- Keto Shrimp Scampi – Chapter

- Zoodles, buttered – Chapter 10

Fish-Lover's Meal

- Keto Fish Nuggets – Chapter 9

- Aioli – Chapter 10

- Keto Rice– Chapter 10

This is just a small sampling of the dishes you can combine to make mouthwatering meals. If you start with these, you can easily mix and match your favorite recipes to create any number of breakfasts, dinners, and suppers. Tweak them to accommodate your nutritional needs. Add your own favorite ingredients and you'll be well on your way to enjoying the ketogenic life.

Conclusion

Now you know how to cook healthier meals for yourself, your family, and your friends that will get your metabolism running high and help you to feel healthy, lose weight, and maintain a balanced diet. A new diet isn't so bad when you have so many options from which to choose. You may miss your carbs, but with all these tasty recipes at your fingertips, you'll find them easily replaced with new favorites.

You will marvel at how much energy you have after sweating though the first week or so of almost no carbs. It can be a challenge, but you can do it! Pretty soon you won't miss those things that bogged down your metabolism and your thinking. You will feel like you can rule the world and do anything, once your body is purged of heavy carbs and you start eating things that rejuvenate your body. It is worth all the detox symptoms when you actually start enjoying the food you are eating and all the incredible benefits that entails.

Now you have everything you need to break free from a dependence on highly processed foods, with all their dangerous additives that your body interprets as toxins. Today, when you want a sandwich for lunch, you'll roll the meat in Swiss cheese or a lettuce leaf and won't miss the bread at all, unless that is, you've made up the Keto Bread recipe you discovered in this book! You can still enjoy your favorite pasta dishes, even taco salad, but without the grogginess in the afternoon that comes with all those unnecessary carbs.

So, energize your life and sustain a healthy body by applying what you've discovered. You don't have to change everything at once. Just start by adopting a new recipe each week that sounds interesting to you. Gradually, swap out less-than-healthy options for ingredients and recipes from this book that will promote your well-being.

Each time you make a healthy substitution or try a new ketogenic recipe, you can feel proud of yourself; you are actually taking good care of your mind and body. Even before you start to experience the benefits of a ketogenic lifestyle, you can feel good because you are choosing the best course for your life. Enjoy.

Thanks for reading. If this book helped you or someone you know in any way, then please spare a few moments right now to leave a nice review.

My Other Books

Be sure to check out my author page at:

USA: https://www.amazon.com/author/susanhollister

UK: http://amzn.to/2qiEzA9

Or simply type my name into the search bar: Susan Hollister

Thank You

Made in the USA
Lexington, KY
26 February 2018